Fine-Tune Your Hormone Symphony

a patient's guide to understanding hormones
and making beautiful music again

1-19-2014

Dear Hyla,

In admiration of

your beautiful music!

So nice to meet you!

Love,

Angeli

NFIM1@bellsouth.net

Angeli Maun Akey, MD, FACP, ABAARM

This publication contains the opinions and ideas of the author. It is intended to provide helpful and informative material on the subjects addressed in the publication. It is sold with the understanding that the author and publisher are not engaged in rendering medical, health, psychological or any other kind of personal professional services in the book alone. The author and publisher specifically disclaim all responsibility for any liability, loss or risk, personal or otherwise, that is incurred as a consequence, directly or indirectly, of the use and application of the contents of this book.

All case studies and testimonials in this book are factual. Where applicable, names and personal information have been omitted for privacy. Each testimonial was approved for use in this book by the respective individual.

Published by Fine Images Printing and Copying
Gainesville, Florida

First published 2011
© 2011 Angeli Maun Akey, MD
All rights reserved.
ISBN 978-1-936634-80-4

No part of this book may be reproduced by any means
in any form without permission in writing by the author.

Credits:
Project editor – Charles R. Hollinger
Assistant Editor – Rosemarie F. Newton, JD, PhD
Graphic Designer – Roy del Castillo
Publisher – Michael Boehlein

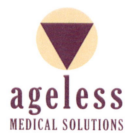

www.agelessmedicalsolutions.com
First Edition

Dedication

This book is dedicated to Tim, Timothy, Jr., and Derek, who keep my conductor healthy and provide a steady stream of oxytocin; To my deceased father, Jesse, who gave me unconditional love; To my mother, Alicia Maun-Martin, MD, who taught me how to treat patients' mind, body, and spirit; To my brother Noel Maun, MD, PhD, who has taught me my whole life but especially in the school of critical and deliberate thinking; To my older sister, Consuelo, who helped me develop the right side of my brain; To my little sister and confidante, Jessica, who always brings fun and laughter; And to my flexible and accommodating staff. And of course, to the many teachers I have had throughout my education, and the thousands of patients who have trusted me with their health and their lives.

"It's good to be a seeker, but sooner or later you have to be a finder. And then it is well to give what you have found, a gift into the world, for whoever will accept it"
    -- *Jonathan Livingston Seagull* by Richard Bach

4

Contents

Introduction	7
Part I: What it takes to feel great	39
How to make beautiful music	
Part II: You, the Conductor	47
A. The Three Angles of Wellness	
B. The Three Spheres of Influence on Personhood	
C. The effects of illness and injury both past and current	
Part III: The Four Sections of the Hormone Symphony	85
A. Strings/ Sex Hormones	
B. Wind/ Metabolism	
C. Percussion/ Thyroid	
D. Brass/ Vitamin D, Parathyroid hormone	
Part IV: Putting It All Together	131
Part V: Plot Your Own Hormone Symphony	141
Conclusion	157
Glossary	159
Appendix	163
Bibliography	167
About the Author	171

6

Introduction

You are reading this book because you don't feel quite the way you used to feel.

You may not know why, but you just don't feel quite right. You remember when you used to feel well, and you want to feel that way again.

I start my new patient visits by asking a simple question: When was the last time you felt GREAT?

People rarely say, "I feel great now." I suspect they would not be in to see me if they felt great. Oftentimes, they know their bodies well enough to know that something is just not right.

A toddler does not know anything about music, but there are certain chord progressions that make sense to the human ear. These chord progressions are rules in the way music moves that are soothing. Wolfgang Amadeus Mozart was a genius at this. That is why when my boys were toddlers crying in the back seat of my Volvo in their car seats, I would put in a Mozart CD, and they would calm right down. There have been some studies that have shown that listening to Mozart helps the young brain to develop in a positive way.

On the other hand, if they heard cacophony such as some heavy metal music or noises that didn't make sense, though they didn't know anything about music and were still nonverbal, they would start to cry.

This book is written for patients and the lay public. You are not expected to know anything about hormones, chemicals and pharmacology, biochemistry or physiology, though that is the science behind what I am teaching you. Like learning the "circle of fifths" or rules for chord progression in writing music, you don't need to know this information to know if the music is good. You don't need to know the science to know when you feel well or not so well.

You know when you feel good. You know intuitively when you are "in tune," and therefore, you know when you are "out of tune." However, you may not be able to describe why you are not feeling so well. Your description of feeling out of tune may be something like this:

I'm tired
I'm burnt out
I can't think straight
I can't remember anything
I am having hot flashes
I'm depressed
I have E.D.
I just don't care anymore
I feel weak when I don't eat
I can't get the tire off my waist
I can't put on the muscle anymore
I can't bounce back from stress
I'm too tired to work out
I don't think about sex
My hair is falling out
I forget   things
My skin   is dry
I can't focus   or concentrate
I don't sleep   well (or at all)

And the litany goes on and on…

(Does this list look like a Rorschach of a big person to you? See Part III B. on metabolic syndrome. Those patients come in with most of the above concerns.)

This step by step guidebook will give you the framework of the basics on feeling well again and managing your "Hormone Symphony."

This model of wellness will help you put how you feel into a "wellness map" which will give you initial guidance for lifestyle and nutritional changes to help your body tune itself. In addition, you will have an idea about which potential part of your hormone systems may need some serious addressing with your physician.

On the inside back cover of this book is my model of the Hormone Symphony. I constructed it three years ago and have used it in my practice since. I have found it an indispensable tool in helping my patients heal, feel well, and play beautiful music again.

The last fold-out page of this book is a simplified version of this model of the Hormone Symphony. You will be filling it out as you progress through this book. Like a "paint by number" picture, you will have a completed roadmap to wellness by the time you make it through this book. So I will call that completed Hormone Symphony picture your "wellness map." I really would encourage you to take the time to fill in the questions that I ask along the way and fill in the last foldout page (in pencil) as you are prompted to do so.

This guidebook will help you tune yourself, the Conductor, and navigate and fine-tune each section of your Hormone Symphony. You will be able to dialogue with your physician when you have completed this book. This wellness map, i.e. the completed simple Hormone Symphony picture, will be like sheet music. It will guide you to playing beautiful music again; it will be your guide to optimal health.

Hormones

It is my observation and belief that **optimization of your hormones is the first line of defense against aging and chronic diseases**. So this is the first place to start in my practice when you are not feeling as well as you used to feel. But it's not just giving you hormones exogenously by prescription but helping your body make the right hormones in the right proportion all by itself. The body wants to heal itself; my studies in other healing traditions helped me understand this. So initially, I help my patients identify and remove the blocks that are causing their bodies to be out of balance. For example, if I have an overweight 35-year-old man with low testosterone, I ask him to lose weight before giving him testosterone replacement because I know that his extra abdominal fat is causing his testosterone to be converted to a female hormone, estradiol. If he eats simple carbohydrates to increase his serotonin levels, then I ask him what is going on in his life that may give him serotonin deficiency. (More on this case later in the book.)

Your optimal health is as individual as your thumbprint

It is my goal for you that you are the best that you can be. Everybody is as unique and different as his or her thumbprints. Everybody has their own DNA and their own health potential. I would like to help you to reach that potential.

Deliberate Aging

Aging is no longer up to chance—you just need assistance in making the optimal aging road map to help you make good choices for your own individual cells. (What might be good for your cells may be harmful to another person's cells, and vice versa.) In addition, I will help you optimize your cellular function.

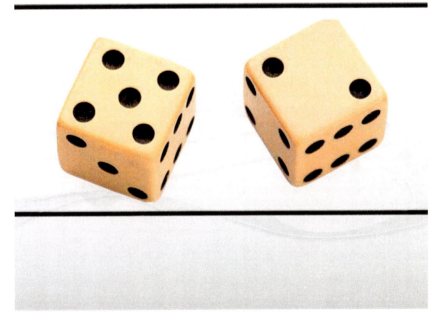

Aging well is no longer by chance. It should not be just a roll of the dice.

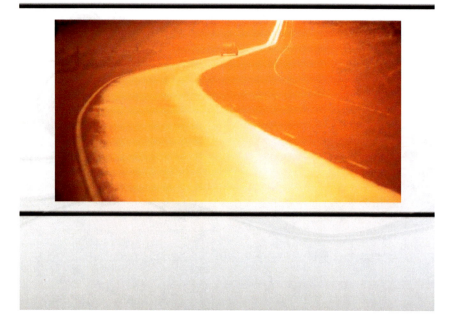

A physician trained in Age Management Medicine can customize an optimal aging road map for you. By the end of this guide, you will have your own personalized wellness map in your completed Hormone Symphony picture located on the last foldout page of this book.

Aging

Aging can be a scary prospect.

One physician, Dr. Eric Braverman, MD, says that aging is a series of pauses—the slowing down of our organ systems (Braverman, 2007). We have all heard of menopause, which is the slowdown of the female reproductive system that comes with big signs like hot flashes and the loss of menstrual periods.

Other "pauses" are subtler. Have you heard of the other pauses like "thyropause"—the slowing down of thyroid function; or "dermatopause"—wrinkling and fragility of skin; or "andropause"—the stage of dropping testosterone levels in men?

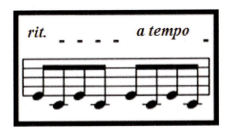

These pauses usually occur after a significant period of *ritardando*, the Italian musical term for slowing down. This is fine if the Conductor is ready to slow down, but if the Conductor wants the tempo to proceed at the current tempo (*a tempo*) but one of the sections of the Hormone Symphony does not acknowledge and starts to retard, then there is discordance. The music does not sound so good, that is, the patient does not feel so well. There is frustration on behalf of the Conductor, and the music does not sound as good as it used to.

Have you felt like that?
Stop now and write down 3 incidences that let you know that your sections are slowing down. These are the reasons you are reading this book.

(For example, "I am gaining fat around my waist," or "I can't recover from my basketball game with the guys like I used to.")

1._____
_____
2._____
_____
3._____
_____

Inflammation and Oxidation

There are basic processes that cause aging to our cells, tissues and organs. The two big ones are inflammation and oxidation.

Inflammation is redness, swelling, pain, tenderness, heat, and disturbed function of an area of the body, especially as a reaction of tissues to injurious agents.

The whole body can be disrupted from an inflammatory diet high in processed white carbohydrates like white bread, pasta, rice and potatoes.

Oxidation is defined as the interaction between oxygen molecules and all the different substances they may contact, from metal to living tissue. However, with the discovery of electrons, oxidation came to be more precisely defined as the loss of at least one electron when two or more substances interact.

When there is a loss of an electron a "free radical" is formed. Free radicals are the result of normal chemical reactions in the body called oxidation which then leaves the body with thousands of unbalanced electrons. These unstable electrons can then cause damage to our cells.

The simplest example of oxidation in metals is rust. Corrosion can occur at a tissue level too. Oxidative stress is involved in pathological processes such as cardiovascular disease and strokes. In essence, during these processes our vessels are "rusting" from the inside out.

When I explained this concept to one of my patients, she made the comment,
"Yeah, Dr. Akey, I'd rather wear out than rust out!"
   --Dorothy, age 62

That is my hope for you, that you tune your Hormone Symphony so well, that you make beautiful music, and that you only wear out from enjoying life to the fullest, instead of rusting from the inside out.

Reaping the benefits of mapping the genome
In addition, we are all programmed with a set of genes that determine our medical future. Just like a computer program, our destiny is in the blueprints to our cells called our DNA. In fact, as a consumer you can order a map of your genes by such commercial labs such as "23 and Me" for about $399 (23 and Me). The report you receive will tell you which illnesses you are at high risk of contracting based on your genes. In the medical literature, the geneticists and ethicists are currently struggling with who is in charge of informing patients about newly discovered gene mutations, and who is in charge of

watching for manifestation of these illnesses—a constantly evolving body of literature. (Wang, McLeod, & Weinshelbaum, 2011) (Bloss, Schork, & Topol, 2011)

There is good news, however.

Based on studies of identical twins, genes are responsible for only about 30% of our future. For example, an autoimmune thyroid disease called Grave's disease has a 35% concordance, lupus has a 25% concordance, and major depression has a 37% concordance among identical twins (Brent, 2008) (Rahman, 2008) (Belmaker, 2008). This means that if one of a set of identical twins has this disorder, then the likelihood of the other in the set having it is the percentage quoted.

In other words, about 70% of the manifestation of the disease state has to do with environmental or other factors. <u>We have the majority of control over our genes!</u> These factors are called "epigenetic" influences. We can manage these epigenetic influences ourselves. Again, the majority of the manifestation of our genes is within our control. If we know first that we have a genetic tendency toward a disease state either by family history or chromosomal mapping, and second, if we are guided on how to modify that gene expression, then we are much better empowered in our health management.

Type 2 Diabetes, a good target for Age Management Medicine

We may be genetically programmed to have, for example, Type 2 diabetes (T2DM), or what has also been called adult-onset diabetes or non-insulin dependent diabetes. This is the type of diabetes where enough insulin is present in the body but the insulin is not interacting or conversing with a cell efficiently.

The key does not fit the lock, so to speak, and so the cell cannot accept the blood sugar floating around in the blood stream. This causes rusting or oxidative stress to the vessels, mostly the tiny little vessels called the arterioles where only one red blood cell passes at a time. This can lead to damage to the small vessels of the eye ("retinopathy") or the small vessels of the kidney ("nephropathy") or the nerves to the feet ("neuropathy").

Nobody wants that, especially those who have the genetic predilection to diabetes based on family history.

If we really have control over the 70% of the environmental factors that determine the physical manifestation of our genes (the phenotypic expression of those genes), then we can modulate them by knowing the epigenetic influences on them. An Age Management Medicine doctor is trained to do this.

The science is there, unlike as recently as even twenty years ago when I started in the medical profession. We now know the risk factors, and how to modify them. In addition, we have science that backs up the plethora of dietary supplements, **nutraceuticals** (see glossary), lifestyle interventions, and medications that can modify the manifestation of the disease state of Type 2 diabetes, for example.

This knowledge is expanding constantly. Thank goodness— because Type 2 diabetes is the medical epidemic of the 21st century in the United States.

In the October 31, 2008 issue of *Morbidity and Mortality Weekly Report*, the Centers for Disease Control and Prevention (CDC) reported that the incidence of new onset Type 2 diabetes in U.S. adults has increased by 90% over the past decade. It is estimated that 1 in 3 adults will have Type 2 diabetes by mid-century. In my section on metabolic syndrome (see Part III: B), the precursor to Type 2 diabetes, you will understand why in the U.S. there is a "perfect storm" for this epidemic.

Type 2 diabetes is not only associated with eye disease and blindness, kidney failure requiring dialysis, loss of feeling in the long nerves causing foot damage which can lead to infections that result in foot amputation (these are the so-called microvascular complications). It is also associated with heart attacks, strokes and peripheral arterial disease (the so-called macrovascular complications).

In medicine we have known about the macrovascular and microvascular complications of Type 2 diabetes for decades. However, there is newly mounting evidence linking Type 2 diabetes to an increased risk for Alzheimer's disease.

The link between Type 2 diabetes and Alzheimer's disease

For 11 years, Japanese researchers followed more than a thousand people, ages 60 and older. Those with Type 2 diabetes at the outset were 35% more likely to develop Alzheimer's. Those with the most severe cases of Type 2 diabetes had more than triple the risk (Ohara, 2011).

The Alzheimer's Association estimates that by mid-century, 16 million Americans could have the disease. Some estimate that one in two of us by age 80 will have Alzheimer's disease.

The fact that Type 2 diabetes is increasing and it's a risk factor for Alzheimer's would only make those numbers bigger.

Why the link between two of America's biggest health problems? Scientists don't have all the answers, but Dr. Sam

Gandy and his team at Mt. Sinai School of Medicine recently discovered one piece of the genetic puzzle.

A team at Mount Sinai Medical School found that the genes that are regulated by insulin also control the build-up of the material in the brain that causes Alzheimer's disease (Lane, 2010).

There are tests like the apoA4 gene test and others that are available to loved ones of a patient stricken with Alzheimer's. However, these are considered specialty labs, costing hundreds of dollars as they are not yet standard coverage by insurance companies. In addition, I am not sure what these data would add to the preventive management I have for a patient whose first-degree relative has Alzheimer's disease because I would consider them high risk and be treating them as such by actively addressing and modifying known epigenetic factors. We already know some of the epigenetic factors in Alzheimer's disease, such as stress. There are studies that show that caretakers of Alzheimer's patients are at higher risk of developing the disease themselves. Also, 20 to 50% of caregivers report symptoms of depression. Some say that depression may be a precursor to dementia.

I have a beautiful couple, both professionals. The husband developed Alzheimer's disease at the peak of his career. It is now a decade later, and she treats him as he progresses with all the tenderness in the world as he wanders around the exam room and can no longer follow simple commands like "open your mouth" when I see them. I tell her that she is a witness to their marriage covenant "to have and to hold, in sickness and in health, 'til death do us part." I enjoy seeing them.

However, I told her that she must take respite care to protect herself from the ravages of the tremendous stress on her

Hormone Symphony, and over the years I have guided her in finding help at night, orchestrating help from their children, making social time with her friends, and continuing her exercise regimen. She asked (for the sake of their children) that I check her husband for the apoA4 gene, which was performed at Mayo clinic. He is indeed positive for the gene. She's not quite sure what she will do with the information, and as of now, hides it from their children. She has relayed to them my recommendations to take high dose fish oils, manage their stress, abstain from alcohol and tobacco, eat organic foods and eat an anti-inflammatory diet like the Mediterranean diet. Other recommendations are to exercise and maintain a good cholesterol profile and lean body weight. I am constantly surveying the medical literature to help them modify the epigenetic factors in prevention of Alzheimer's disease as they are identified.

It is estimated that the body of medical knowledge doubles every four years

Medical science is expanding rapidly. It is estimated that every four years we double our medical knowledge as a whole. If these estimates are correct, during the next four years we will learn as much about medicine as was discovered from the beginning of human existence until now. This is mind-boggling to me, akin to studying our ever-expanding universe in astronomy, just in the opposite direction – going inward instead of outward. I believe science is just uncovering what is already there, and it is so exciting!

We have so much knowledge now, that we need to study and standardize the basic method by which we obtain, refine, extend and apply that knowledge. This has affected medical education as well. When I graduated from medical school in

1993, the emphasis was on knowledge—memorizing facts and applying facts.

I remember as a 3rd year medical student at the University of Florida, my shoulder became sore because I used to carry around a 6-pound, 4-inch thick *Harrison's Textbook of Internal Medicine* on my internal medicine hospital rotation. My older sister had sewn for me a custom holder for that book so I carried it around the wards like a heavy purse. I was working my way through the whole book and found it a great joy to find a patient and then find within the volume which condition he/she had and read about it.

As I teach the third year medical students now, a much more expansive, electronic knowledge base is about two seconds away at all times. They carry more on their smart phones than the large volume I carried on my shoulder, and with a lot less strain on their musculoskeletal system!

So, I tell them on day one of a rotation with me that they will not be evaluated on knowledge, because that is as easy as turning on their computer or portable device. I tell them I will be evaluating them on their ability to communicate with the patient enough to frame a clinical question. With this as a starting point, I expect them to do the research and implement the answer in an intervention that takes into account the framework of knowing the patient as an individual.

Then when the answers to the clinical question are found through research, I watch how the medical student interacts with the patient in prioritizing and coming up with a mutually agreed upon treatment plan. Without the understanding and "buy-in" of the patient, great treatment plans are useless. So, I teach the medical students this Hormone Symphony model which promotes understanding and buy-in from the patient perspective, thereby increasing compliance. My patients are getting excellent results and my medical students feel much more confident in their doctor-patient relationships.

Figuring out how to manage and apply all of the information is an enormous challenge, one made even more complex by <u>biochemical individuality</u>: the fact that each of us is unique. In both preventive medicine and traditional curative medicine, what works well for most people may have adverse effects on any given individual—thus, the limitation of the gold standard in clinical research, the "double-blind, placebo-controlled, clinical trial." Many interventions are not considered validated for this reason. Over the past decade, the National Institutes of Health has established the National Center for Complementary and Alternative Medicine (NCCAM), which is scientifically validating ancient treatments like acupuncture for back pain, and rejecting other CAM interventions that did not work when subjected to rigorous scientific analysis.

However, most clinical research is still being funded by industry, the pharmaceutical companies. Like any other business, there has to be a return on investment (ROI), and in the United States, it takes millions of dollars to have a drug approved by the Food and Drug Administration (FDA). It's much easier in Europe or Asia to have a drug go from the research bench to the public. While I think that in most cases this kind of safety is a good thing, it also means that only drugs with the potential for millions of dollars to the pharmaceutical company have a chance of having an extensive rigorous clinical trial—one sufficient to bring it to the consumers in the United States.

Interventions that have little to no return on investment will probably not be studied. For example, I have heard and tried and seen improvement with the use of Vicks VapoRub™ applied topically to toenail fungus twice daily for twelve weeks with trimming back of the nails. No one will invest in this trial because the ROI is not there. Yet by clinical observation, many of us practitioners have noted improvement with this intervention. Physiologically it makes sense as the eucalyptus may be changing the pH of the toenail making it less inhabitable to the fungus. I do not think it's harmful but potentially helpful to my patients, and it is a lot less costly than the approximately $60 prescription topical medication I used to prescribe, which had variable results. So, I am going to continue to recommend it.

There are many other types of alternative medicine herbs or interventions that have been simply labeled as "not studied." In reality, it means that no one has found the clinical question worth investing in; this means there are many non-validated medical interventions because no one has invested in research for them! When I suspect that an intervention is useful based on physiology and biochemistry, and as long as it's not harmful, I am usually willing to investigate it and try it with my patients. I tell them that there isn't much data on trying a certain herb or intervention, and we review what available data there is and then we make decisions together. For example, the use of ground up chia seeds in lowering cholesterol has as much data as the use of oatmeal. It has fiber, antioxidants, and is a food with potentially medicinal properties, so I recommend it.

Hopefully, the new science of human genomics will really help us individualize medical interventions. We are already starting to see the beginnings of this type of customized medicine. For example, take the MTHFR gene mutation, which is associated with **methylation**. Methylation is a biochemical process that is associated with detoxification and is needed in the formation of chemical messengers in the brain called "neurotransmitters." I look for this gene mutation in families with recalcitrant depression or in my "migraineurs," or patients that suffer with migraine headaches. The treatment is simple: it's methylated folic acid. Many people buy folic acid that is not methylated, but people with the MTHFR gene mutation are unable to use the non-methylated type of folic acid. A simple intervention of methylated folic acid can help these people with depression and migraines. The pharmaceutical industry figured this out with their studies on prescription strength methylated folic acid called DEPLIN™. It was initially marketed as an antidepressant, but when the insurance companies paying for these medications realized it was just methylated folic acid, they quit covering it under psychiatric coverage so that they wouldn't have to pay for it, AND it was re-classified as a medical food.

If you want to read more about how our health care system has been controlled and sometimes undermined by our pharmaceutical industry, read Marcia Angell's book, *The Truth About the Drug Companies* (2004). She is the previous editor of the prestigious medical journal, *The New England Journal of Medicine*, and Harvard-affiliated.

What to expect from an Age Management Medicine physician specialist

Your physician specializing in Age Management Medicine is your best ally in the fight against chronic diseases.

Such a physician is trained to:
  a. Keep up with the rapidly changing knowledge base in medical science as it applies to prevention
  b. Identify the very earliest footprints of chronic disease at the pre-symptomatic phase
  c. Identify interventions to delay the onset of that disease or at least slow down its progression
  d. Trained to apply interventions prudently, based on physiology and biochemistry and without the undue bias of pharmaceutical companies

The Hormone Symphony

From philosopher Hans Urs Von Balthasar of the early 1900s, who said that "truth is symphonic," to theologian Fr. Thomas Dubay who said that "truth is the symphony of beauty," came the late physician Dr. John Lee, who coined the term "Hormone Symphony."

Dr. John Lee was one of the founding fathers of bioidentical hormones who used the idea of the symphony in explaining the human body, which made a lot of sense to me. Both a symphony and the human body are complex, yet sound simple and beautiful when performing well.

About three years ago, I created my model of the Hormone Symphony to teach my patients about how their bodies work and to develop treatment plans they will support. Often these include exercise and diet prescriptions, sleep prescriptions, nutritional supplements, deletion of harmful lifestyle habits, and bioidentical hormones.

What I have found is that when a patient understands why I have asked them to do what they are doing, or which part of the Hormone Symphony is being affected, we not only have a basis for dialogue but also I have found patients empowered to execute the treatment plan in the context of their lives. Alternatively, I ask them to be frank with me during the visit and tell me if they feel treatment recommendation is overwhelming, in which case I know to break the plan down into stages.

This book is designed to help you discover which part(s) of your Hormone Symphony need to be tuned. With the information that you will have compiled by being an active participant as you work through this book, you will have a working agenda to review with your physician. You, the Conductor, must take control of your health. Ultimately, _you_ are responsible for your own health. Hopefully your physician will be open to the discussion and order appropriate biochemical testing and intervention if he/she thinks them appropriate. Your physician should be your ally in tuning your Hormone Symphony and making beautiful music again.

So let's get started...

Like any good symphony, your body has a conductor and four main orchestra sections (hormone types).

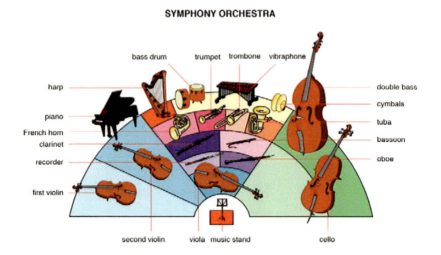

A musical symphony has a conductor and four main sections. The sections are the strings, wind, percussion, and brass.

Like a true musical symphony, the most important member is the conductor and YOU are the Conductor of your Hormone Symphony.

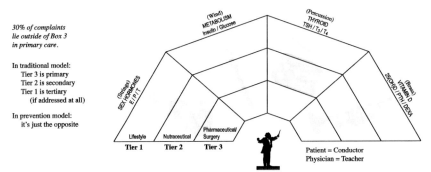

The above diagram is located on the inside back cover of this book so that you can write on it. Note, like the "chairs" of a musical symphony, the "first chair" is usually the best instrumentalist within the section; the "second chair" is the second best, and the "third chair" is the third best instrumentalist. In the Hormone Symphony, I have three tiers of intervention.

In my model of Hormone Symphony, the best intervention, the first tier intervention is lifestyle, the second tier intervention is nutrition/nutraceutical supplementation, and the third tier intervention is pharmaceutical medication/surgery.

In the traditional curative medical model, tier 3 interventions of pharmaceutical drugs and surgery are often the only ones discussed. I think there are multiple reasons for this, including medical training and time constraints, but it is a suboptimal approach.

Note that the (+) is the list of recommendations to help the particular section of the symphony. For example, try now plotting (in pencil) on the lifestyle (+) section of the Strings section, "HIIT training" into slot 4a (see Appendix A...more on HIIT training later). It would look like this:

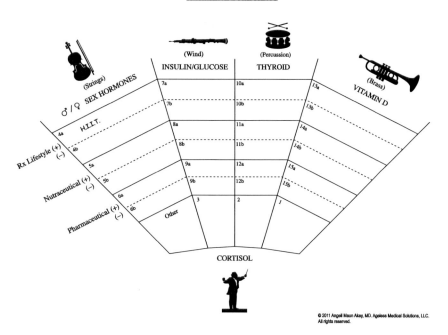

On the other hand, if fasting glucose was high, to help the Wind section (metabolism), removal of simple carbohydrates like white bread, pasta, rice and potatoes in the diet to optimize the insulin/glucose interaction would be the first order of business. It would be plotted on the lifestyle (-) section into slot 7b and look like this:

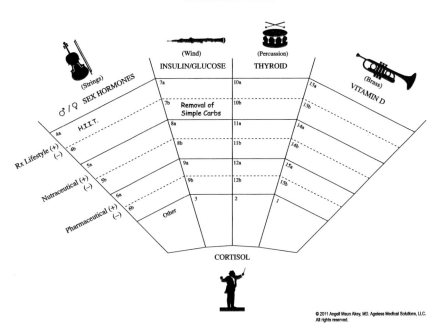

Now, the analogies:

Conductor	You, the patient	Meaning	Hormones
Strings	Sex Hormones	Love	Testosterone, estrogen, progesterone
Wind	Metabolism	Energy	Insulin, glucose (hemoglobin A1C)
Percussion	Thyroid	Rhythm	Thyroid stimulating hormone, Free T4, Free T3
Brass	Vitamin D	Structure	25 –hydroxy Vitamin D, calcium, parathyroid hormone (PTH)

You, the conductor of the Hormone Symphony

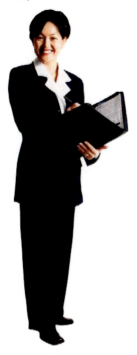

If you are balanced and well, "healthy," it means your Hormone Symphony is playing in tune.

If you (as the Conductor) are not well, no matter how well the individual sections of the Hormone Symphony can play, the music is not what it should be. The symphony cannot play properly without the Conductor.

I spent the first ten years of my clinical practice "tuning" the sections of the Hormone Symphony, making sure the numbers on the labs were just right. For example, I would make sure that my patients with diabetes had a hemoglobin A1C under 7 mmol/mol, or that their TSH was optimized at about 1 µIU/mL. Please do not worry about those terms, just realize that doctors use numbers and laboratory data to guide how we are doing in chronic disease management. In fact, the insurance companies and now the federal government use these numbers to evaluate physician competence. These numbers are used to report "outcome measures."

But I began to realize that no matter how well I tuned the sections of the Hormone Symphony—that is, making sure the numbers of the sex hormones, the metabolism, the thyroid and my treatment of bone health were just right—if the person (the Conductor) was not right, they still didn't feel well. In other words, the music was still "out of tune."

Take for example, Vivaldi's "Four Seasons" symphony. I particularly like this symphony because its four movements of Spring, Summer, Fall, and Winter parallel the metaphorical stages of life. If I attended a concert and the music was beautiful during the Spring movement, but at the beginning of Summer movement the conductor fell sick with a migraine headache and tried to push through the Summer movement anyway, the music probably would not be as beautiful as it would have been had the conductor been healthy. Note that the sections of the musical symphony didn't change; they are still in tune, but not as tuned as they had been to each other because the conductor was not up to par. The flow became disrupted. In other words, the conductor has to be healthy and in touch with the sections to make optimally beautiful music and create balanced harmony - that is the difference between and good performance and a <u>GREAT</u> performance.

You know what I am talking about if you have ever been to a concert of any type. In my experience, when the "flow" is happening everything seems so effortless, and I am transported to another place and time. That is why I like music so much and why I like the symphony metaphor to teach this approach. Music breaks down language barriers and is the voice of the soul. Thus, this Hormone Symphony model will require some serious "soul-searching."

In the second decade of my practice, I started studying the person. I have become as much a humanist as a scientist. I suppose that is why Hippocrates said "medicine owes the art of clinical inspection and observation."

When I began to see my patients from a three-dimensional view AND tune the Hormone Symphony, they started becoming dramatically better.

Care of the Conductor (You)
Dr. Mehmet Oz and colleagues recently published a series of health books called "You: The Owner's Manual," on basic care of the human body. This is a topic that should be taught from kindergarten on up. Further, it's a difficult battle to be healthy and have healthful habits because our society seems rigged against it. In many ways, our society stacks the odds against healthy living.

Activity
We average 4,000 steps in our daily activities, but the Centers for Disease Control and Prevention recommends that our minimum daily requirement for activity be 10,000 steps. That is equivalent to about five miles per day. People in other nations have to walk this much to get to their jobs, grocery

stores, and run errands. This is equivalent to about 30 to 60 minutes of walking depending on the pace. If my patient is logging 10,000 steps, and I recommend a pedometer for measurement, and weight loss is still not occurring, then I recommend increasing the plan by 2,500 steps (which is equivalent to about one mile and about a 100-Kcal expenditure for a 150 pound person).

In addition, Americans have a "do it yesterday" mentality, which drives up stress and cortisol levels. We may be more industrious than many other nations, but we pay a terrible price. And, unfortunately, we are now a video and internet-centered culture, and much of this involves sitting for long periods.

Nutrition

The standard American diet (ironically called the "SAD" diet) is mostly processed, high in animal fat and unhealthy fat (saturated, hydrogenated fat), and low in fiber and complex carbohydrates. There are many epidemiological studies that show that this type of diet increases risk for cancer, heart disease, stroke, and intestinal disorders like colon cancer.

In my opinion, the real "SAD" part about this is that we in the United States actually can afford to eat foods that are just the opposite, foods that <u>decrease</u> risk for chronic disease. Specifically, the way we should eat should be low in saturated, hydrogenated fats, and high in plant-based foods that increase fiber and complex carbohydrates.

Americans average 2.1 servings of fruits and vegetables combined daily. You may have heard of the goal of 5 fruit and vegetable servings combined daily, but even that is too little.

The Center for Science in the Public Interest has recommended for years that we eat 5-9 servings per day. The American Institute for Cancer Research is so convinced of the cancer-fighting abilities of fruits and vegetables that they have been recommending 9-11 servings each day. The 2005 federal guidelines call for as many as 13 half-cup servings of fruits and vegetables per day.

There are other decisions to face when making food choices. We now have the burden of avoiding genetically modified foods here in the United States. The Pew Initiative on Food and Biotechnology in 2004 reported that 45% of corn, 85% of soybeans and 76% of cotton in the United States was genetically modified. I suspect this may have something to do with the current explosion of gluten sensitivity and other food sensitivities. In fact, the European Union (EU) has banned many genetically modified foods that we produce in the United States.

Try to eat whole foods, plant-based and organic (which automatically means non-genetically modified), with proteins primarily being low-mercury wild fish and white lean poultry (preferably free-range chicken or turkey not given hormones).

I tell my patients we need to go back to eating like Laura Ingalls Wilder in *Little House on the Prairie* (the 1800s). Remember how it took Ma all day to make a meal and Laura would go fishing with her sisters and they would shuck their own corn and harvest their own greens?

Also, it's important to drink enough water. A good rule of thumb is to drink one ounce for every kilogram of body weight (and increase water consumption while exercising).

Lastly, you need 20 minutes of non-peak sun exposure per day. That means avoid the sun between 10 a.m. and 2 p.m. If you care about wrinkles, you may want to cover up your face and décolletage and expose your arms and legs. Sun exposure will help convert your Vitamin D to active form.

Part I: What it takes to feel great

How to make beautiful music

40

CASE STUDY: "Out of Tune"

Vivian is a 49-year-old equine champion and mother of three girls, who came to me for feelings of depression, hot flashes, insomnia, and "just not feeling like myself." Her vitality with her family and her horses was just not there anymore.

"I have insomnia, I wasn't able to lose the last 10 pounds since my last child, I have a depression like I've never gone through before, I have irregular periods, hot flashes and no interest in my husband. I tire easily," she said.

What she was really saying was:
"HELP, I'm out of TUNE!"

Examine the chart:

Statement	Part of Hormone Symphony	Section	Hormones
"insomnia"	Conductor Strings Percussion	adrenal/ sex hormones/thyroid	Cortisol/DHEA, E/P/T TSH
"not able to lose last 10 pounds"	Wind	metabolism	Insulin (glucose)
"depression"	Conductor Strings Percussion, Brass, Wind (all sections)	All sections	All hormones
"irregular periods, hot flashes, low libido"	Strings	Sex hormones	E/P/T
"tire easily" fatigue	All sections	All sections	All hormones
"I just didn't feel like myself at all"	All sections	All sections	All hormones

Case Analysis

Just like when my infant sons would recognize when the music wasn't good or melodious and soothing, but would calm right down when a Mozart CD was played, all of us intuitively know when we feel good and healthy and when we are not feeling very well.

Sometimes a state of depletion (incurred by insomnia caused by the perimenopausal transition such as in Vivian's), sets off a cascade of events that leads the Hormone Symphony to playing discordant sounds. She was fatigued and easily irritable. She and her family recognized this.

She came to see me for the obvious—the Strings section (sex hormones) was out of tune. This is what most women come in for. With personality changes being much more subtle than changes in something physical (like menstrual length and flow), it's not surprising. In the process, this lead to a detailed analysis of her Conductor which included shoring up her basic good habits of nutrition, and encouraging her horseback riding time, which gave her both exercise and a meditative state.

She had also expressed desire to engage in her previous spirituality practices that had been placed on the back burner with raising children, and I encouraged that (Box 1). We evaluated her Three Spheres of Influence (Box 2) and she voiced her concern about her children growing older and the expenses over the horses she enjoyed so well. I told her that she was worth having horses and besides, they gave her the opportunity for meditation (calming her stress), and gave her a wonderful opportunity for exercise. Actually, some of my fittest patients are horse enthusiasts. Between mucking stalls and riding, they have the three types of fitness that I emphasize [cardiopulmonary training with HIIT (see Appendix A), resistance and core training, and balance training (Box 1)]. I encouraged her to continue to develop her own identity apart from her all-encompassing role as mother at this stage in her life, especially as she moves steadily toward "empty nest syndrome."

Like most women in the perimenopausal transition (who are facing the "empty nest syndrome" in the next few years), I encouraged that she re-develop a strong friendship and intimacy with her husband. Usually when the youngest child is in 9th grade, I tell both my male and female patients the importance of dialogue so that feelings can be openly shared and losses related to aging can be mourned together. I tell my patients that the relationship will not be the same relationship they shared prior to children; that would be impossible. But, it has the potential to be even better—on a level of intimacy far beyond the physical needs of a man and woman in their 20s that often brought them together in the first place.

This evaluation of self is never easy. Any growth phase I liken to labor and delivery, it's a birthing process with all of the pain and tears. However, the prize in the end is worth it.

Much of her emotional strain had to do with physical depletion from lack of deep, restful sleep. Sleep and rejuvenating the Conductor was the first order of business. I recommended melatonin 3mg up to 15mg, with L- theanine 200mg at night to block the early morning stress-related awakenings. Just achieving a great night of sleep put her on the road to recovery.

Then, I tuned the Strings section with bioidentical hormones, and as I found osteopenia (early weakening of the bones), I tuned the Brass section with Vitamin D, calcium and a weight bearing program.

The results were tremendous. She was able to sleep again, she was interested in her horses again, she lost twelve pounds, the fatigue was gone, and she paid me the best compliment when she said "my husband wants to send you flowers." Yes, the music was in tune again in Vivian's house.

Case Conclusion

So what does it take to feel great? How does beautiful music sound? It's all about balance and harmony. It's different for every individual, as different as their DNA and the epigenetic factors affecting their DNA. But the overarching theme to feeling great and making beautiful music is balance and harmony. That's true of the Hormone Symphony.

For example, if the Percussion section is too strong compared to the rest of the symphony (like in Grave's disease, where an autoimmune process causes release of too much thyroid hormone), then the Hormone Symphony is not excellent. With Grave's disease, the patient cannot sleep, has running mental thoughts, muscle weakness, tremor, unintentional weight loss, and diarrhea. The other hormones are overrun by the thyroid hormones. To have this Hormone Symphony tuned, the thyroid section has to be turned down to balance the rest through medications and sometimes radiation of the thyroid gland.

Have you ever been to a concert where the drums, the percussion, were so loud, it felt like your ears were going to burst? Yet without the rhythm section, something would be lost in the music. So the key is <u>balance</u>.

Chinese culture emphasizes balance. From their martial arts forms, to Chinese medicine, to herbal medicine, to balancing the foods on their plate between "hot foods" and "cold foods,"-- it's about balance.

I, too, believe it's balance that allows us to play beautiful music for all to hear and enjoy. We have this music in us and it is unique to us individually. As a physician, scientist, humanist, and musician, I really do believe it's the balance of mind-body-spirituality that allows us to play the unique, beautiful music that is inside of us for all to hear and enjoy.

When this complete view of a person is recognized and validated, there is a tremendous healing force now engaged in the treatment plan.

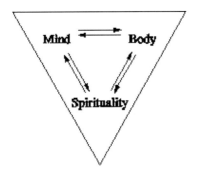

Part II: You, the Conductor

    A. The Three Angles of Wellness
    B. The Three Spheres of Influence on Personhood
    C. The effects of illness and injury, both past and current

48

Part II: A. The Three Angles of Wellness

This is my form of asking the doctor's standard "Social History" and "Review of Symptoms".

There are three angles that must be addressed in the lifestyle of you, the Conductor. As in Chinese medicine, I believe that there is always a force and an opposing force, and these plus the net balance of all the other forces equal the health of the Conductor. The yin-yang effect of life forces is not static, it is dynamic. Always, there is a tendency to entropy, a basic law in physics, for all things to have a tendency to disorder. The best way to counter this is with will. The good news is that you can re-order your health and make beautiful music. The decision is yours. Take control of your Hormone Symphony.

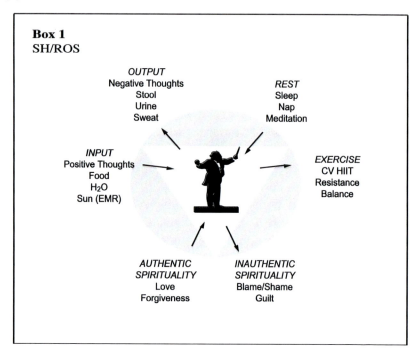

Angle 1: Focus on the Mind

1. Inputs – at a very basic level, the four inputs that affect us every day are thoughts, food, water and radiation (including the sun and electronics)
2. Outputs – we emit thoughts, stool, urine and sweat/detoxification; I recommend these occur at least daily

Angle 2: Focus on the Body

1. Rest – there are different types of rest, physical rest in the form of naps or sleep, and mental rest in the form of meditation and prayer

2. Exercise – the three types of exercise that I emphasize are cardiovascular exercise, specifically HIIT (high-intensity interval training) also known as PACE (progressively accelerated cardiovascular exercise) training, resistance training, and balance; I think that all three are necessary in optimal aging

Angle 3: Focus on Spirituality
1. Spirituality – any spirituality that leads to love and forgiveness is energizing
2. Inauthentic spirituality is destructive, oftentimes involving blame/shame and guilt

In youth, these basic Three Angles of Wellness can often be ignored or not done at all, and health can be maintained. However, with each passing year, they become more and more important in the care of you, the Conductor. The tendency towards entropy becomes more pronounced with aging; the peak of our health is age 35. After that, one has to exercise more and eat less just to maintain the same health as the previous year, and the ability to handle stress diminishes. Focusing on the mind and on the body is effective in healing, but I find it incomplete. Especially in difficult times, one needs to go beyond one's self and reach out to a higher power and include authentic spirituality in the healing process. Remember that <u>authentic spirituality</u> is the kind that leads to love and forgiveness, and heals all aspects of life. Inauthentic spirituality leads to blame/shame and guilt and is destructive (see Box 1).

More on spirituality

Authentic spirituality is often needed because, as the saying goes, "to err is human, to forgive is divine." As a doctor, I have been privy to stories of the most treacherous and unspeakable violations of what a human can inflict on another human. From infidelity to molestation to incest to rape to attempted murder, I have held my patients' hands (both men and women) as they would speak the unspeakable. I am truly blessed to be trusted with the stories of such pain. I do not think it possible to forgive such treachery by human will alone. I believe it involves supernatural grace. I ask the ones that have experienced such horror, yet now are balanced, healthy, and making beautiful music how it is possible. It seems that all of these well-adjusted people tell me the same thing, "I forgave them by the grace of God."

From my own experience, I have found that <u>forgiveness is a decision</u> and the first step to starting the healing process. As a first year medical student, my father was involved in a non-fatal car accident. He was taken to an affiliated hospital where he died at age 54 of a <u>simple medical error</u>—not from his wounds sustained in the car accident. I was angry, confused and bitter. I wanted to drop out of medical school. In fact, I did take a leave of a couple of months. The anger was eating me up alive. How could the hospital where I would be training in my later years kill my father? The "what if's" kept me up at night; I was stressed and could not sleep at all. My father was the "wind beneath my wings" up to that point in my life and he was taken away in a very unjust way, I felt. What added insult to injury was that it happened in an affiliated hospital where I was studying to be a doctor! Eventually, my family, my priest, and my medical school advisors talked me into going back to medical school. But, I can honestly say that I had to specifically forgive the surgical resident that missed accessing my dad's airway that night of the accident before I could start the process of healing and moving forward. From my own experience, this only happened "by the grace of God."

Now the resident that missed my dad's airway had no intention of doing so, it was a real accident. I have observed in my patients that being the intentional victim of another's evil intentions could be a lot more painful and the process of forgiveness and healing can be much more difficult. From a health perspective, though, I am convinced still that forgiveness has to be the first step. From what I have seen, through the grace of God, "all things are possible" (Matthew 19:26, NAB), even forgiveness for such horror. I also recall the passage from Ephesians "All bitterness, fury, anger, shouting, and reviling must be removed from you, along with all malice. [And] be kind to one another, compassionate, forgiving one another as God has forgiven you in Christ" (Ephesians 4:31-32, NAB). (For more on forgiveness of malice, read the novel *The Shack* by William Paul Young.)

I have come to the conclusion through such personal experiences and through observation of patients through twenty years in medicine that blame/shame, guilt, anger, and resentment are major roadblocks to healing even on a physical level. Lack of forgiveness is like drinking poison and hoping the other person dies.

Thankfully, I believe the opposite is also true. <u>I believe that love and forgiveness engages an incomprehensible healing force and sometimes true physical healing occurs, but always an emotional and spiritual healing happens.</u>

This is an area of active research in an area of medicine called psycho-neuro-immunology (or how the psyche of a person affects the brain which can affect the immune system). See the reference on malignant melanoma patients who participated in group psychotherapy shortly after their diagnosis showing enhanced immunological functioning after six months versus the control group who did not engage in group psychotherapy, cited in Part II: C. of this book.

Part II: B. The Three Spheres of Influence on Personhood

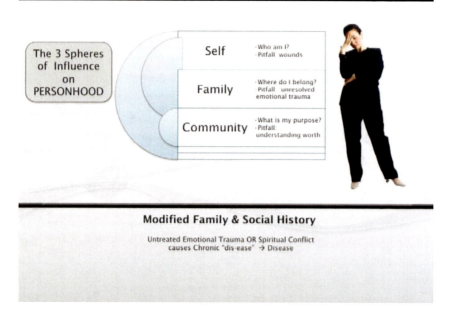

The Three Spheres of Influence on Personhood: Self, Family, and Community

This actually is my form of a doctor's standard "Family History" and "Social History. " Family of origin plays an important role in the subsequent health of the individual (Peck, 1978). It is impossible to dissect out mind from body.

Unresolved emotional wounds from childhood lead to chronic "dis-EASE" which can lead to chronic disease. Some have hypothesized this to be the case with a hormonally mediated female condition called endometriosis.

The excessive stress of a childhood trauma can disrupt the subsequent balance of female hormones with the net result of "estrogen dominance," in which too much estrogen in relation to progesterone causes excessive amount of endometrial tissue to grow. (Endometrial tissue is the inner lining of the uterus where a fertilized egg can implant.) Endometriosis occurs when these cells actually migrate out to the pelvic cavity, seeding areas where they do not belong (like the colon and the fallopian tube), which leads to very severe pain during menstrual periods, and potentially infertility.

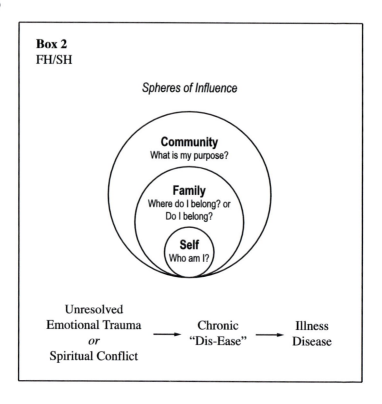

1. SELF: Who am I?

Over the ages, the greatest philosophers and theologians have grappled with this question, and a detailed discussion is beyond the scope of this book.

However, it is important that each of us understands that we are loved unconditionally and that we are important, so that we may have foundational "self-esteem."

Many of my patients that have physical illnesses often have not explored the question of "who am I?" or if they have, they have concluded in a negative way that they are not worth anything, that they are garbage. With a negative self-image, it's hard to move forward. The core of who we are is the basic building block on which the total self can be erected; it's foundational, and a healthy self-image or positive self-esteem is critical to physical health. I believe that not only our neurotransmitters and hormones work better with this state of mind, but the lifestyle changes that I recommend are more likely to be implemented and maintained with this foundational building block of a positive self-esteem.

Many times there are childhood wounds that have left this foundation cracked. Perhaps an early childhood divorce of parents has subconsciously left the child blaming his/herself for their parents' failed marriage.

Perhaps there was early childhood abuse from an alcoholic parent, be it sexual or physical or emotional. Maybe there was relentless teasing for being overweight, or having a funny nose or floppy ears. Decades later, these "childhood wounds" can result in broken adults.

Fill-in Questions:
1. My childhood overall was _____ (describe with one word).
2. On a scale of one to ten with one being minimal and ten being maximal, I would rate this overall feeling a _____.
3. If I could go back and change one thing about my childhood it would be:
   _____
   _____
   _____.
4. I will now reflect privately, with love and understanding (without writing them down) on the people who have wronged me. I choose to forgive them now.

2. FAMILY: Where do I belong?

It is important that we feel like we belong somewhere.

Human beings by nature are social creatures; we first learn how to interact within our family of origin, who provide us with tendencies in our personalities. We learn how to cope, and even learn the **masks** that we wear in day-to-day living. Masks are neither good nor bad—they help us navigate in society.

Sometimes, however, these disguises are worn too tightly, often a result of unresolved emotional trauma as a child. They can get in the way of true intimacy and lead to loneliness. It is my belief that we have to be our true authentic self, at least in front of one other person, so as to bask and grow in the unconditional love of that other, like a plant grows toward sunlight. John Powell's books are most helpful in understanding unconditional love in the development of self (Powell, 1967, 1969, 1974, 1978).

There are basic types of masks that help us to function in society as grown-ups. Though these masks may serve a good purpose, they affect all our relationships to some degree. Masks define our personalities, but can also negatively affect others' disposition to us. Most people have one default mask, but may change it depending on who they are with.

Which mask(s) do you wear?

Mask	Description	Pitfall
Clown	Always laughing	Uncomfortable with serious topics
Congenial	Always Agreeable	Denial of self
Superman/ Wonder-woman	"Yes, I can do everything"	Sets expectations too high; stress
Martyr	Takes and performs responsibilities through guilt or for approval	Burn-out, bitterness, resentment
Controller	Gets things done; gives orders	Unable to see good qualities in others, inhibits growth in others, always makes decisions for others
Calm/ Cool/ Collected	Mr. or Mrs. Cool, self-possessed	Stifles or denies feelings of others
Bulldozer	Agenda takes priority; controls conversation	Overwhelms / inundates others; can ignore their feelings
Mr. or Mrs. Clean	Cleanliness in environment is basis of self-esteem	Anxiety develops with disorder, can impair relationships
Insecure/poor self-image	Totally focused on his/her limitations	Infantile superficial relationships based on dependence
Hypochondriac	Gets attention through illness/ aches or pains real or perceived	Can result in real illness; cry-wolf effect

Mask	Description	Pitfall
Mr. or Mrs. People Pleaser	Gets attention through unconditional service	Sacrifice to the detriment of self
Cynic/Pessimist/Nihilist	Criticizes others; pretends to not care/believe	Afraid of self-investment; doesn't take risks; can't commit fully
Hero/Messiah	Rescues others; attracted to flawed people	Unhealthy relationships/tries to fix people; pet and material hoarding; instead of mutual relationships, has parental relationships
Narcissist/Egotist	Excessive self-confidence in appearance and abilities/traits	Overwhelming to others; vanity/pride; feels entitled to more than others; spoiled
Perfectionist	Always has to be perfect every time; Nothing less is acceptable	Perpetually unsatisfied; causes anxiety to oneself and those around him/her, prone to depression and negativity

Fill-in Questions:
1. My main mask is _____
2. The ways I use my mask are _____
   _____
   _____

3. My mask serves me in the following ways (name 3):
   _____
   _____
   _____

4. I can comfortably take my mask off in front of these people:_____
   _____

3. COMMUNITY: What is my purpose?

This is the final and most important of life's questions. Purpose is the reason we get up in the morning. Everybody, from the very young to the very old, needs to feel needed, purposeful, and loved.

When we feel like we are not fulfilling our purpose, there is great inner conflict. People are gifted with talents—they are the music inside of us. It's in the discovery of these talents and finding ways to use them in a purposeful way that leads us to feel like we are living a purposeful life. This is the key to playing a beautiful Hormone Symphony. The definition of purpose varies with each individual. The process of self-discovery is the process of discovering purpose.

One obstacle to understanding purpose is a feeling of worth that is tied to material or physical success. With unemployment reaching 10%, that leaves many Americans very vulnerable to feelings of worthlessness. I explain to my patients who have recently lost jobs, especially the males in my practice, that their worth is not tied to their employment. I encourage them to take inventory of what other aspects of their lives besides employment make them worthwhile. I explain to them that their worth is intrinsic and not tied to any one THING outside of themselves. I encourage them to go to Scripture (both the Hebrew Bible and New Testament) for much evidence of this.

Answer these questions:
1. What unique talents or abilities do I have? (list top 3)
   _____
   _____
   _____

2. How am I using these talents in a purposeful way?
   _____
   _____
   _____

3. What is my purpose?
   _____
   _____
   _____

Life's Three Great Questions

Sphere of Influence	Question	Lack of clarity results in:
Self (Self Esteem)	***Who am I?***	Confusion
Family (Identity)	***Where do I belong, or do I belong at all?***	Lack of security, lack of grounding
Community (Purpose)	***What is my purpose?***	Listlessness, feelings of unworthiness, unsettled.

Summary:
The answers to these three of life's great questions often take a lifetime of discovery. These questions and progressive answers outlined in life stages are best delineated, in my opinion, by Dr. Carl Jung, a medical doctor and psychiatrist at the turn of the 20th century. A contemporary of Sigmund Freud, I find Dr. Jung's work much more user-friendly. He outlines the progressive maturity of a person in various life stages.

Becoming fully human and fully alive: From adolescence to adulthood

"An unexamined life is not worth living."
    -- Socrates

Life's three great questions answered in an affirmative manner results in an individual who is fully human and fully alive, an emotionally well-balanced person with clear purpose. From a Jungian perspective, this person has advanced from adolescence to adulthood. This person can make beautiful music. Stop now and think of the people in your life that make such beautiful music. Most likely they have explored and answered life's three great questions for themselves. Their Conductor is standing firmly on Box 2. They know who they are, where they belong and what their purpose is. They have found foundational self-esteem.

However, the only permanent thing in life is change. Life is dynamic. Even these people have movement in their Box 1, 2, or 3. However, they always seem to reach an equilibrium or homeostasis again. Especially in Box 2, I have found that when at least two of the Three Spheres of Influence are moving, or have major activity, there is much turmoil in my patients' lives. It can lead to a state of anxiety or depression. It is very common in my clinical practice to find this, and I point out to my patient that it is like they are in the phase of labor in birthing a child. It's very painful, but the growth at the other end of the pain is very beautiful like seeing the baby after a long labor process and painful delivery. All of my moms understand this. The dads understand this too, especially those who have seen their wives through the birthing process.

Another analogy is like the maturation of a caterpillar in a cocoon. As it develops and squeezes and dries out, it eventually becomes a beautiful butterfly, but there are no shortcuts. If one were to try to cut the cocoon open before the caterpillar is mature enough to become a butterfly, it would die. Its wings are not yet ready to fly.

CASE STUDY: "Late Adolescence"

It seems to me that we can stay in the stage of adolescence for an inordinate amount of time. I have many patients, mostly females in their 50s and early 60s, who come in stressed and anxious because their 80- or 90-year-old mother still controls them. The patient cannot seem to please her mother, and she is at the same time anxious and angry. I point out that she has never clearly differentiated herself from her mother and thus she is still trapped in the stage of adolescence. Oftentimes when I bring this up to the patient, a light bulb of understanding goes on and the patient can move forward realizing that she does not have to react passively anymore. When the daggers of abusive words are thrown, they can instead be deflected with love and will no longer hurt. This rebellion usually happens during the teen years, but may not happen until the 50s or 60s. I ask her to understand that her mother probably did the best that she could, the best that she knew how—that her mother is/was only human. This leads to liberation, especially when I ask my patient to look at her mother with eyes of tenderness, love, and forgiveness.

Sphere of Influence	Question	Clarity results in
Self (defines self-esteem)	Who am I?	Positive Self-Esteem
Family (defines identity)	Where do I belong? Or Do I belong?	Security and stability
Community (defines purpose)	What is my purpose?	Clear feelings of worth

So, can you answer the following?
(Remember any one of these can take a lifetime to answer, so take heart and start, the attempt itself is an act of courage.)

Who am I?
_____
_____
_____

Where do I belong (or do I belong)?
_____
_____
_____

What is my purpose?
_____
_____
_____

I believe that untreated emotional trauma and/or spiritual conflict (lack of forgiveness, harbored anger, and guilt or blame/shame), lead to chronic dis-EASE [discomfort] and later chronic disease, a full physical manifestation of internal emotional states. This, I truly believe, is the mind affecting the body's physiology, or mind over matter in a negative sense.

True examples of this that I have witnessed in clinical practice:

- A 23-year-old man who had a heart-wrenching breakup that included infidelity and a reversal of personality of his girlfriend (to a substance-abusing, sinister person), which left him sleep-deprived and severely depressed for several years. After having little to no success with almost every antidepressant prescribed by other doctors, he came to see me for tertiary hypogonadism—which had caused brain fog, a 30-pound weight gain, low energy, and low libido.

(Tertiary hypogonadism is where the hypothalamus, the hormone control center of the brain, is suppressed and not producing hormones to tell the pituitary gland in the brain to release hormones to tell the testicles to produce testosterone.)

- A 47-year-old woman receives a diagnosis of breast cancer and then stops menstruating that month.

- A 67-year-old mother (whose son does research in the Andes) finds out he is lost, and her metabolic syndrome converts to full blown Type 2 diabetes.

SUMMARY

Sphere of Influence	Defines	Question	Lack of clarity results in	Clarity results in
Self	Self-esteem	Who am I?	Confusion	Positive self-esteem
Family	Identity	Where do I belong?	Insecurity, instability	Security and stability
Community	Worth	What is my purpose?	Listlessness, feelings of unworthiness, unsettled feelings	Clear feelings of worth

Part II: C. The effects of illness and injury, both past and current

Here is some food for thought:

"Sixty-one percent of all primary care clients surveyed and 69% of depressed clients desired counseling, but relatively few desired a referral to a mental health specialist."
-D. Brody et al., *"Patients' perspectives on the management of emotional distress in primary care settings,"* **General Internal Medicine**, 1997, Jul 12 (7).

"Among primary care clients with major depression, disabling chronic pain was present in 41% of those with major depression versus 10% of those without it."
-Bruce Arnow, *"Comorbid Depression, Chronic Pain, and Disability in Primary Care."* **Psychosomatic Medicine**, 2006, 68.

"Seven of the ten leading causes of death (heart disease, cancer, stroke, chronic lower respiratory disease, accidents, diabetes and suicide) have a psychological and/or behavioral component."
-**CDC**, 2005.

"Malignant melanoma patients who participated in group psychotherapy shortly after their diagnosis showed more enhanced immunological functioning after six months than did a similar group of melanoma patients who did not engage in group psychotherapy."
-F. Fawzy. *"Malignant melanoma: Effects of an early structured psychiatric intervention, coping, and affective state on recurrence and survival 6 years later."* **Archives of General Psychiatry,** 1993, 50.

"In a study of emergency room patients with chest pain, nearly 41% met criteria for either an anxiety or depressive disorder as a primary medical diagnosis."
-K.Yingling, **General Internal Medicine,** 1993, 8.

"Primary care clients experiencing physical symptoms with a possible psychosocial component (e.g., palpitations, gastrointestinal disturbances, headaches, malaise, and sleep disorders) were randomly assigned to either behavioral interventions using didactic material, relaxation-response training, awareness training, and cognitive restructuring or to treatment focusing on information about stress management and its relation to illness. At six months, clients in the behavioral groups showed significantly greater reductions in medical visits and in discomfort from physical and psychological symptoms than did the clients in the information group."
-CJ Hellman, *"A study of the effectiveness of two group behavioral medicine interventions for patients with psychosomatic complaints."* **Behavioral Medicine,** *1990, 16(4).*

It is important to know that only 70% of medical complaints or concerns are found in the physical realm in an adult primary care practice like mine. The rest are found elsewhere as evidenced above. In other words, in only 70% of visits to a primary care physician's office can the determination of the concern be found to be physical (like an abnormal chest X-ray, blood work, or physical exam).

Advanced training in my internal medicine residency has made me an aggressive diagnostician. But when everything physical has been ruled out, the thirty percent of concerns left over are called "functional illnesses."

> **Box 3**
> Current Illness/PMH/PSH
>
> *70% of primary care complaints here*
>
> Acute Illness
>
> Chronic Disease
>
> Past Surgical History
>
> Past Trauma History
> (physical or emotional)

For example, in polite medical language for the chart, the doctor would write, "I did the complete work-up for this patient's abdominal pain (CT scans, colonoscopy, endoscopy, biopsies, blood work), and all were normal. Therefore she has a functional GI illness."

This is doctor-speak for "this lady is crazy, I did the 'million-dollar work-up' and I can't find anything." I used to say this myself, as the diagnostic tools and equipment and training that I had about ten years ago had been all I could go by. When we in medicine have reached our therapeutic ceiling, we tend to blame the patient. In the chart, this may read "supra-tentorial" or "psycho-somatic" or "somatization" type of illness.

However, in broadening my vista to include other types of healing including Chinese medicine and acupuncture and methods like "pulse diagnosis" and understanding energy channel or "meridians," and studying herbology and Ayurvedic medicine and now Age Management Medicine, it's rare that I find that I don't have a therapeutic plan to offer my patients.

I am able to develop such a plan because of exposure to different healing traditions. I am grateful that I do this with my base of an Ivy-League residency training in internal medicine at Yale University; and solid, basic medical science degrees from the University of Florida with undergraduate college degrees in music and interdisciplinary science, and an MD from the University of Florida College of Medicine Junior Honors Medical Program. The Junior Honors Medical Program taught me how to read very challenging scientific literature.

Without this perspective, I believe that I would be bored and frustrated in my current practice of primary care internal medicine. I say "practice" because medicine is always changing. It really does take a lot of practice, I learn from my patients every single day. I teach my students to have an attitude of a lifetime of learning. Every day, one has to keep up with the reading and questioning.

It is rare that I have a dull day. I believe that science is discovering what is already there. With the risk of sounding overly theological or philosophical, it's from this basis that my mind is open to the limitless opportunities and healing traditions that are available.

In fact, I find what I do extremely stimulating and rewarding. Physician means teacher, and I enjoy teaching. From teaching the medical students to teaching patients and my staff, to using the oldest in diagnostic descriptions of energy found in the meridians, to using the latest in diagnostic tests, I find medicine and the healing profession to be like a perpetually expanding universe.

In other words, how exactly my patients heal is not as important to me as the fact that they can in fact heal. It used to bother me if I did not understand the sequence of events that caused the healing to occur. Always, I try to search this out to learn for the next patient. However, sometimes healing just happens—in these cases, it is mysterious and unexplainable by science. Thus, I have accepted that these do happen, and have collected many stories of prayer and healing that will be published soon in a book that is being written concurrently with this one entitled, *A Referral to the Divine Physician*.

The "Art" of Medicine
Twenty years into my vocation as a physician, I am convinced that many times the healing comes simply in the exam room as I intently listen to the deepest part of a patient's beating heart.

That's the "art" of medicine.

CASE STUDY: "The Mind Controlling the Matter"
Just last month, a patient came to see me for menopausal hormone management. In the discussion I reviewed the Three Spheres of Influence. When I asked her directly about childhood trauma, the conversation came to an abrupt pause as tears welled up in her eyes.

She stutteringly said, "Dr. Akey, when I was four years old, my cousin sexually abused me. My mom did not believe me, and so I suppressed it, thinking it didn't happen. You are the first person since then that I have shared this with."

I sat there stunned, calculating that as she was 49 years old, she had kept this locked inside for 45 years. I acknowledged how painful the experience must have been for her. Then she started crying as a flood of emotion started to come forth as from a burst dam. I gave her a hug as she trembled like the four-year-old girl who didn't get affirmation from her mother. Maybe at that point, God was using me to be that affirmation she had so longed for 45 years ago.

As I looked at her with the eyes of a physician, with her morbid obesity, her four medications for anxious depression, her six medications for metabolic syndrome, and her stressful high-powered job, it all made sense to me.

Case Analysis
This one traumatic event in the life of a 4-year-old child, defined this lady for the rest of her life. I would suspect that with affirmation and protection instead of rejection from her mother, life would have been totally different for her. She would have been much healthier physically.

My treatment plan therefore would <u>not</u> focus on her morbid obesity, her back pain, her metabolic syndrome, nor her anxious depression; my treatment plan would focus on forgiveness of her mother, her cousin, herself (children internalize blame with lack of information), and developing her self-esteem. She needed a referral to a professional therapist. From my observation sometimes trauma can be processed more quickly with medications, but rarely can it be completely healed without counseling. I use psychologists trained in a type of trauma healing called **EMDR** (Eye Movement Desensitization and Reprocessing). It does not involve drugs or hypnosis. It is a simple technique that has the patient talk about his/her trauma while following the therapist's hand movements, or a moving light. The result is that the patient "processes" trauma much more quickly. I have witnessed an EMDR session with one of my patients, and it seems that the memory becomes repackaged such that the constant stimulation to the adrenal glands caused by the trauma gets cut off. I have found this is very effective with deep traumas.

Like an abscess the body walled off so the patient does not go into fatal septic shock (but still causes symptoms such as low grade fever, aches and pains and fatigue), severe but deeply buried emotional trauma may show itself in other dysfunctions. These need to be uncovered and addressed. However, healing for this type of trauma has to be done with a well-trained compassionate therapist, as he/she is treading on very tender parts of the human spirit. I liken it to doing fine microscopic vascular surgery—precision and utmost care must be exercised by the therapist. In surgical treatment of an abscess, there is an initial opening of the wound which brings major relief but the wound itself takes time to completely heal during which time the patient will experience discomfort.

The same is true for deep emotional wounds that are opened through processes such as EMDR. It's not for the faint of heart for either the patient or therapist, and can take weeks to months to years to complete the process. However, from what I have witnessed, like labor and delivery, the pain is worth it in the end. These patients that successfully traverse the pain of opening these wounds and healing are now liberated. They are now free to make beautiful music with their Hormone Symphony.

Case Conclusion: The Three Spheres of Influence

In using the model of the Three Spheres of Influence from the previous chapter (Self, Family, and Community), this is how I would plot this patient's emotional "self-talk" (in bold) and what that confrontation with her mother at 4 years of age did to her:

Sphere of Influence:	Defines your	Question	Lack of clarity results in	Clarity results in
Self	Self-esteem	Who am I?	**"Mommy doesn't believe me"** =Confusion, poor self esteem	Positive self-esteem
Family	Identity	Where do I belong?	**"Mommy did not stand up for me"** =Insecurity, instability	Security and stability
Community	Worth	What is my purpose?	**"I must be unlovable"** =Feelings of listlessness, unworthiness, non-closure	Clear feelings of worth

On the other hand, if the patient's mom would have listened to her and backed her up in this difficult situation at 4 years of age, instead of being too afraid to "rock the boat" of the family, the outcome would have been much different. It probably would have looked like the following, and there would have been clarity instead of a lack thereof. The patient's plot of The Three Spheres of Influence would have looked much more positive, as seen here (in bold):

Sphere of Influence	Defines	Question	Lack of Clarity Results in	Clarity results in
Self	Self-esteem	Who am I?	"Mommy doesn't believe I am telling the truth" = Confusion, poor self esteem	*"Mommy believes me, and will protect and stick up for me. I am worth sticking up for"* =Positive self-esteem
Family	Identity	Where do I belong?	"Mommy did not stand up for me" =Insecurity, instability	*"Mommy loves me enough to risk her own place in her family structure to stick up for me"* =Security
Community	Worth	What is my purpose?	"I must be unlovable." =Listlessness, feelings of unworthiness, unsettled feelings	*"I must be worth a lot to Mommy, I have unconditional love and acceptance"* =Clear feelings of worth

As you can see from the chart, one action many years ago could have started a negative chain of events in the patient's health, affecting her almost fifty years later. This revelation during the interview was extremely important. Once I explained this to her, she was silent for several moments. I could see that she was struggling with a mixture of strong emotions as she searched for the right words.

I could then tell she had a feeling of great relief and acceptance. She then understood why she had difficulty in her intimate relationships and why she had three failed marriages, difficulty mothering her daughters (but not her sons), difficulty letting her "Controller" mask down for anybody, and has never been emotionally intimate with anyone.

I told her that her mother had let her down, that her process of healing would be to release the blame and shame of the event—specifically the blame of her mother for not affirming her and the shame she felt associated with the event of abuse. I told her that forgiveness is a process—she must choose to forgive but it's OK not to forget (though I asked her to let go of the associated negative feelings with the event). I told her eventually she would have to confront and forgive her now 62-year-old cousin. I told her from a health perspective that lack of forgiveness is like her drinking poison and hoping the other person (her cousin) dies. I believed that her cousin has no memory of the event and an event that affected her and her physiology the rest of her life is probably completely out of his consciousness, perhaps even since that day.

I felt the cathartic nature of this discussion was probably enough for a day's visit (and better suited for a therapist trained in EMDR), so we moved on to list her current illnesses, pertinent past medical history and surgical history, and other past trauma. Essentially we went into the "Past Medical and Surgical History" part of the interview which we are taught in medical school. My method, however, is designed to be much more in depth and critical in understanding the person.

These are the questions I ask:
(Refer to Box 3 on the inside back cover)

1. What are your current symptoms?
2. Have these symptoms been given labels in the past?
3. Do you have any chronic disease (like rheumatoid arthritis, diabetes mellitus type 2 or adult onset diabetes)?
4. How do these chronic diseases impact you and your lifestyle?
5. Past surgical history?
6. Do any of these past surgeries still impact you? (for example after gallbladder removal, it is common to have "dumping syndrome" where eating fatty food can result in a rapid trip to the bathroom with diarrhea, or back surgery like laminectomy failing and leaving one with chronic low back pain.)
7. If these medical or surgical illnesses still affect you, rate and label them for severity (0 being no impact, 10 being the highest level of impact on your life).
8. Past trauma history:
   Have you been involved in any trauma in your life? For example, car accidents, concussions from sport injuries, falls, military, or trauma inflicted by another—either physically, sexually, spiritually, emotionally?
   Have you ever been touched in an uncomfortable way by someone you know?
9. How is this trauma affecting you now? In other words, do you have chronic pain, sleepless nights, or nightmares, or pent up anger that's been unexpressed or unacknowledged?
10. Do you feel safe and happy at home?

CASE STUDY: "Running on Empty"
DEPLETION versus DEPRESSION and "Adrenal Fatigue"

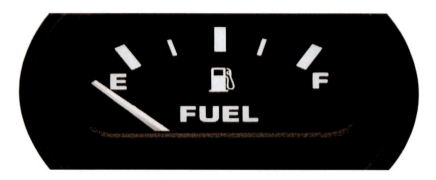

Ann, a 41-year-old mother of two who works two jobs, tries to keep her house clean, exercises, and has a type A personality. She wears the mask of the "Perfectionist" and "People Pleaser," being the third child of four. She wants to appear to the world that she has everything under control, and it seems like she did until these past two years when everything seemed harder, including her menstrual periods. Her husband says that her PMS is so severe, he schedules business trips away from town during that time of the month. During her premenstrual phases, she craves salt and sugar and favors McDonald's™ French fries dipped in their ice cream. She is frustrated with her expanding waistline. For the past two months she has been up at night with tooth pain that has been undiagnosed by the dentist.

One day she snaps. She feels like she has had enough, she is tired, cannot arise out of bed in the morning, and doesn't look forward to going to work. Nothing brings her joy anymore. She cannot stand her husband and finds coming home after work to a messy house and her children's homework overwhelming. She's easily tearful and explains that she just wants to run away.

Case Analysis

I wish that taking care of human beings would be as easy as prescribing a medication. With traditional primary care internal medicine visits running about fifteen minutes, sometimes I feel like I am drowning in a litany of patient concerns and the time constraints stresses my own Conductor. I suspect that the insurance companies that have caused the average outpatient internal medicine visit to be fifteen minutes think it's as easy as "here's your drug, get out of my office, okay then, next patient." For this patient, about ten years ago, I may have prescribed Prozac™ and a referral to a psychotherapist— that would have been a fifteen minute visit!

But now that I know better, I cannot with a clear conscience do that. It wouldn't serve this patient long term. Frankly, for me it would take away the joy of serving my patients because I would know deep in my heart that I did not do what was absolutely best for that patient.

When I hear symptoms of depression on my annual physical questionnaire such as:
"I feel hopeless and helpless," "I do not look forward to the future," or "I cannot sleep because I am anxious," I have to delve in more deeply.

Certainly there are cases of biochemical depression with long family histories of depression. For these I check gene mutations such as the MTHFR gene mutation, which is associated with kindred families of recalcitrant depression.

Know, however, that there is a fine line between depression and DEPLETION. Our rush-rush-rush society and poor nutrition and lack of exercise have left us a setup for a depleted physical state. When this happens, we may actually feel depressed and wonder "where did my get up and go, GO?" This may be depletion (Body/physical) and not depression (Mind/mental).

When this happens, I hear descriptions that the world looks black and white and no longer colorful. Essentially this patient has lost his/her luster for life. I do a simple litmus test for depletion. I tell this type of person to go on vacation (a real vacation—no cell phones, no computers or internet, preferably no television as the news can be very stressful) for a week and see if the mood changes. If that person returns back to vigor and vitality with the time off and decreased stress, he/she is primarily depleted, not depressed.

I always evaluate sleep patterns. The easiest way to make the Conductor sick is to take his/her sleep away. Sleep apnea is commonly diagnosed in my practice, especially with the burgeoning of obesity. But in Ann's case, her sleep disruption was from pain. She was coping until the tooth pain kept her up for many nights and the lack of solid sleep became the proverbial "straw that broke the camel's back."

Also, too often nowadays people sacrifice sleep in favor of getting more work done or pursuing their hobbies—burning the midnight oil. But if done regularly it can become unhealthy.

Poor sleep makes you fat
In fact, without sleep, cortisol levels go up, as does craving for salt and sugar. A recent study published in the *Archives of Internal Medicine* reported that the ratios of newly discovered appetite hormones that control feeding (leptin and ghrelin) change unfavorably with poor sleep as well.

"Research subjects who slept only four hours a night for two nights had an 18 percent decrease in leptin, a hormone that tells the brain there is no need for more food, and a 28 percent increase in ghrelin, a hormone that triggers hunger" (Spiegel, 2004).

The net effect is hunger (just remember that **leptin** = fullness, **ghrelin** = hunger).

Thus, lack of sleep will not only urge you to eat unhealthy salty and sugary foods through increased cortisol levels; it will also make you eat more because of higher ghrelin and lower leptin levels! I tell patients to remember that ghrelin is the "gremlin" that makes you hungry.

In addition, I will do four point cortisol curves through saliva testing throughout the day (8 a.m., 12 noon, 4 p.m. and 8 p.m.) which most accurately defines how the adrenal glands are functioning in real-time throughout the day. This is based on data from NASA, and is still used to evaluate the health status of their pilots. A normal healthy cortisol curve looks like a ski jump curve—high in the morning at 8 a.m. and then a slowly and gently decreasing slope throughout the day until its low enough at bedtime, so restful sleep can occur. For this patient, the cortisol curves were above normal—she had elevated cortisol patterns from the pain and stress of not sleeping. No wonder she was on edge!

It makes logical sense that a morning blood test for cortisol would not give the whole picture. Firstly, it is only one data point in time. Secondly, if I request you fast all night and then have the phlebotomist stick you with a needle, the stress levels would be high simply from the stress of fasting and then the pain of the needle, so you expect a higher blood cortisol level.

Also, I have questionnaires to screen for excessive adrenal stress, casually termed "adrenal fatigue." More appropriately this is described as "hypoadrenia" (low adrenal function) or "hyperadrenia" (high adrenal function). In both conditions, cortisol levels are still within the norm but not considered optimal for health. In medical school, I only learned about total adrenal failure called "Addison's disease," most often autoimmune (where the body attacks its own adrenal gland); or in the intensive care unit, the adrenal glands bleed into themselves under severe and life-threatening stress, such as overwhelming blood infection. This is called "Friedrich-Waterhouse syndrome." On the other hand, markedly excessive cortisol levels (caused by an adrenal tumor making excessive cortisol) is called "Cushing's syndrome." We were taught to look for a buffalo hump (fat pad at the nape of the neck) and abdominal striae (lines on the abdomen from excessive growth and fat), and high blood sugars. Also, if I had a patient given excessive or prolonged prednisone (a steroid drug to decrease inflammation) I would look to see if they developed "Cushingoid" features—features that looked like Cushing's syndrome but were caused by medication. These people look puffy and edematous. That's all I was taught about the adrenal glands.

However, in my clinical practice, I have seen the ravages of stress on the body and this can best be related to adrenal function. Oftentimes, as with this patient with hyperadrenia, patients complain of insomnia, irritability (short fuses), salt and sugar craving, fatigue, and gaining weight around the waist.

When the saliva tests are plotted, they are above the normal curves but not pathologic to the level of Cushing's syndrome. The patient describes themselves as being "wired and wired" or "wired and tired." They often are driving themselves with caffeine, salt and sugar. Their energy is artificially derived through caffeine—coffee, diet sodas, energy drinks, and sugary snacks. This is not what nature intended. It's not surprising that coffee and donuts are the classic fare for the 10 a.m. and 3 p.m. "coffee break," when there is a natural lull in cortisol. However, this is like putting your foot on the gas and the breaks of your car at the same time. We all know from driver's education class that we will burn out the brake pads and the motor of the car.

Similarly, left alone, with this amount of stress and stimulants used to keep on going, this "wired and tired" person starts to crash, "burn out," and eventually no amount of stimulants can drive this person to have energy and function. Stimulants finally lose all effectiveness and the person is in a never ending spiral of perpetual fatigue. They are "tired and tired."

What is the time course of this? I have observed it is variable. This can go on for months to years before the patient starts to crash. They "burn – out" so to speak, and you can see this in the salivary cortisol curves plotted throughout the day where eventually the salivary cortisol curves look flat. Sometimes, I meet these patients after they have had a litany of illnesses and psychiatric diagnoses. Oftentimes they have seen dozens of doctors prior and are on a <u>dozen or more</u> prescription medications. I am their last hope, because they are so physically dysfunctional that they are thinking about applying for medical disability. These patients come with the diagnosis of "major depression," "anxiety," "chronic fatigue syndrome," or "fibromyalgia." These people are no longer "wired and tired," they are "tired and tired."

Case Conclusion

First, it was critical to balance this patient's entire symphony starting with the Conductor, the basic care of herself, including nutrition, exercise, and sleep patterns (Box 1). Second, I asked her to take off the "Perfectionist" and "People Pleaser" mask, and deal with the resentment she had of her husband. Third, she had residual issues to resolve with her mom as she transitions from adolescence to adulthood in her life stages (Box 2). Fourth, she needed to find the source of her mouth pain. I changed her dentist. The new dentist discovered two occult cracked teeth and repaired them, alleviating her nocturnal pain so she could sleep without pain (Box 3). Also, to address her adrenal issues (the Conductor), I incorporated RITM SCENAR™ biofeedback treatment protocols to help her relax at night. RITM SCENAR™ is a medical biofeedback device that has an FDA registration for relaxation training and FDA clearance for pain management (Tarakanov, 2003). Finally, she needed some progesterone as she is in the Premenopause (see next chapter), to balance the Strings section of her symphony.

These are my medical mysteries. Many times there is an underlying problem that set them up for abnormal cortisol curves like undiagnosed food sensitivities and "leaky gut," or unresolved childhood trauma like sexual abuse, or undiagnosed chronic infection, or type A personalities (like Ann, they often wear the mask of "Perfectionism," which drives the adrenal glands). The treatment plan is extensive and I liken it to undoing a knotted up delicate gold necklace—we have to uncover and undo one knot at a time.

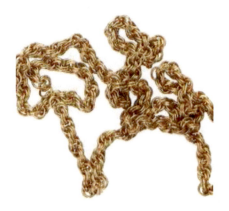

Part III: The Four Sections of the Hormone Symphony

   A. Strings/ Sex Hormones
      1. Menopause
      2. Andropause
   B. Wind/ Metabolism
   C. Percussion/ Thyroid
   D. Brass/ Vitamin D, Parathyroid hormone

The Sections of the Hormone Symphony

"Happiness is not a matter of intensity but of balance, order, rhythm and harmony".
    --Thomas Merton

Now that the Conductor is understood from multiple dimensions (traditionally in medical school language, we would have covered the "Past Medical History, the Past Surgical History, the Family History, the Social History and the Review of Symptoms" in a very unique and thorough fashion where the patient feels understood), we are now ready to cover the sections of the Hormone Symphony.

Oftentimes, it's actually the sections of the Hormone Symphony that brings a patient to my office. For example, if a patient says "I'm having hot flashes," it is either from estrogen withdrawal, the Strings section of the Hormone Symphony (sex hormones) or from excessive adrenal stress (the Conductor).

If my patient says, "I cannot lose weight around my belly," I know to look at stress and sleep patterns (the Conductor), the Wind section (metabolism), the Percussion section (thyroid), and the Brass section (Vitamin D).

Part III: A. Strings/Sex Hormones

The sex steroid hormones affect every cell in the body. My boys are pre-teens and from their development of male body odor, to the deepening of their voices, new acne, their sprouting height, to the newly rough way that they play, it is obvious that testosterone is working on every one of their cells.

It wasn't that long ago that they were not much different than their female counterparts in class. Now with both sexes producing their hormones and emitting pheromones, there is a definite awkwardness that has developed in their classrooms.

Both men and women have a combination of estrogen, progesterone, and testosterone. There are others, but for simplicity, I will focus on these three.

There are subtypes of each hormone. For example, the three main estrogens that are discussed in treatment with "bioidentical hormones" are estradiol (the strongest estrogen), estriol, and estrone (Files, 2011). There are subtypes of androgens such as testosterone and DHEA.

One differentiation that I must make is between natural progesterone, which is what the body knows and makes, and a "progestin," which is a synthetic form. Both are considered in the class of hormones called progestogen (named for this class of hormone's role in maintaining pregnancy, i.e. pro-gestational). It is the synthetic progestogens called "progestins" that might increase breast cancer risk. Unfortunately, all birth controls containing progestogens have only the synthetic kind, the progestins. American studies on birth control have focused on the decreased risk of ovarian cancer due to decreased frequency of ovulation since birth control decreases frequency of ovulation.

It is interesting to note that when progestogens are used to support fertility, the infertility specialists or reproductive endocrinologists <u>only use bioidentical progesterone</u>, not synthetic progestins. So why is it ok to expose non-pregnant women to synthetic progestins?

Both men and women have estrogen, progesterone, and testosterone, just in different ratios. As a premenopausal woman, I have about one tenth of my husband's testosterone level. He has about one tenth of my estrogen levels.

However, after menopause and with andropause (or male aging associated with decreased testosterone levels), that can actually reverse. More on that later.

Simplified table of functions of the 3 main hormones:

Hormone	Brain function	Body effects	Lack of hormone causes:	Too much causes:
Estrogen	Acts as a serotonin reuptake inhibitor, dopamine agonist (like the mechanism of some anti-depressants)	Grows breasts, hips, buttocks, gets the body ready for childbearing, grows the uterine lining	Hot flashes, depression, memory loss	Estrogen dominance (see Strings chapter)
Progesterone	GABA effects on brain, relaxation (like alcohol); receptors found on coronary arteries	Counters effects of estrogen, sheds the lining of the uterus, pronounced at the 2nd half or luteal phase of the menstrual cycle	Anxiety, insomnia	Ovarian cysts, discordant menstrual cycles
Testosterone	Brain effects: confidence to aggression (adolescent boys and risky behavior)	Libido in both men and women, lean muscle mass, unfavorable effect on lipid profile, potential increase of heart disease	Depression, fatigue, insomnia, lack luster view on life, body fat, memory loss	Aggression hyper-sexuality, acne

You see, relative levels of estrogen, progesterone, and testosterone affect every cell in the body. At different stages in life, there may be aberrancy in the relative values of each. You may have heard of the following:

- Male babies being born with protuberant nipple buds from high maternal estrogen in utero.

- Women with polycystic ovarian syndrome (PCOS). These are patients with excessive amounts of insulin associated with excessive amounts of male hormones (like testosterone) causing facial hair and acne and body types that look un-feminizing (lack of waist, fat pad on upper back). Oftentimes this can be greatly corrected by dropping insulin levels by eating a diet rich in vegetables and protein (less refined carbohydrates) and insulin-sensitizing nutraceutical supplementation.

- Men with excessively large abdomens consistent with metabolic syndrome (Santa Claus physique), often have large breasts and small testicles and impotence. This is because the abdominal fat converts their testosterone to estrogen. They often have higher estrogen levels than their menopausal wives!

Let me explain further how a man can even start <u>appearing</u> more female than his wife. If his wife goes through menopause without her hormones adjusted/ replaced, she starts losing her breasts from lack of estrogen, her ovaries start to fall asleep so her hormones are now made in the adrenal glands which may make more male hormones causing features like coarsening of the face and whiskers (yes whiskers!). She gains the average twenty pounds transitioning menopause so her previous hour glass shape becomes linear and she may start appearing more masculine than her husband. At the same time, due to his excessive belly fat, he is converting his declining testosterone levels to estrogen, so he is developing smaller testicles and larger breasts! This is what I mean when I said that in the menopause/andropause phase of a couple's life, he may actually look more female than his wife (but she may start resembling how he used to look)!

WOMEN

Besides the menarche when menstruation starts, and its irregularity for the first few years, the transitions in usual female hormones patterns start to occur around age 35. Classically, at age 35, the progesterone starts dropping leading to conditions of estrogen dominance such as premenstrual syndrome (PMS), weight gain, and fibrocystic breasts. At about age 40, the testosterone starts dropping and my patients complain that they have decreasing libido (Davis, 2008). They also tell me that their husbands somehow look less attractive to them, they have difficulty with sexual climax and orgasm, fat accumulation (especially around the waist), and loss of their mental "edge." Also, sometimes this comes with new emotional states, like feelings of less confidence, and anxiety/depression. Finally, in the mid to late 40s, the estrogen levels start to drop and this can cause hot flashes, poor sleep, memory problems, and vaginal dryness. There are many variations on this theme, like a piece of music, but this is the general direction of how female hormones change.

Menopause

Menopause is defined as the complete cessation of menstrual periods for twelve consecutive months. The average American woman goes through menopause at age 51.

However, the period leading up to menopause has been variably named. I will go with Dr. John Lee's definition of that period (Lee, 2006).

Perimenopause

Perimenopause means "right around menopause," the year or two before, during, or after menstrual cycles end. Cycles and mood are irregular. I often manage this with oral bioidentical progesterone and mood calming nutraceutical supplements as well as melatonin and L-theanine to help my patients to sleep. Also I recommend plenty of exercise, good nutrition, stress management and sleep.

Premenopause

However, the Premenopause can begin as early as the mid-30s. If you are a woman between 30 and 50, you may have PMS, fibroids or benign tumors of the uterus, fibrocystic or lumpy breasts, weight gain, fatigue, irritability, mood swings, bleeding between periods, migraine headaches (especially related to the menstrual cycle and bleeding), water retention, memory loss, or cold hands and feet. This is often exacerbated by stress—which is often driven by our American attitude and lifestyle which drives cortisol.

Here's how: it's thought that the above is created by an imbalance in the ratio of estrogen to progesterone called "estrogen dominance." This is worsened by stress because the stress hormone, called cortisol, steals progesterone which counters the effects of estrogen. In other words, cortisol disrupts this balance. I have heard this referred to as "progesterone steal" at some medical meetings.

Women sometimes come to see me with severe Premenopause symptoms that are exacerbated by stress; for example, severe PMS (premenstrual syndrome) and PMDD (premenstrual dysphoric disorder). These can cause equal dysfunction or disruption in family life. However, these can markedly diminish when these women are less stressed, like while on vacation. These women are often wearing the masks of "Superwoman" or the "Controller" or "Mrs. Clean."

I don't think the era that I grew up in the post women's lib generation [I was born in 1970] was helpful at all to women's health and hormones. I value the fact that women have made it in the workplace (though there is still discrepancy in pay), but I believe that the mental drive encapsulated by that awful jingle for Enjoli™ perfume in the 1970s was terribly wrong.

Remember it? The words were:
♫ *I can bring home the bacon, fry it up in a pan, and never, ever let you forget you're a man, because I'm a woman... Enjoli™.* ♫

Well, my name is similar (Angeli), and from my own life experience, I know that this is not physiologically possible. The message to my generation of women was downright wrong.

I am a working mom with two medical practices, a husband, and two boys ages 11 and 12. I can tell you that after seeing a full day of primary care patients, I have no interest in making dinner, cleaning my house, or having sex!

The best I can do is run about the block three times with our dog Trooper and do 10 push-ups and 10 sit-ups so I don't feel like a hypocrite when I see patients the next day and instruct them to do high intensity interval training (HIIT) and some resistance training. Then I eat dinner that my awesome husband Tim has made, ask the boys how school went and sometimes help with their homework, take a shower, write medical charts, and fall asleep. That's it.

So, I tell my patients that we were sold a bill of goods when we were told "you can have it all" (work, children, and great sex-life) left over from the 1960s. They forgot to tell us the last half of that: "just not all at the same time." So, I encourage my premenopausal patients, like I have taught myself, to be more kind and gentle with ourselves.

Let me repeat that message. I believe that we women can have it all but not all at the same time. We need to decrease our stress levels so that our hormones can balance, so that we can make beautiful music. We have to be kind and gentle with ourselves. We have to realize that not one size fits all and that life is in flux.

Some days our work may demand more of us, some days the children's homework may demand more of us, some days our relationships with our husbands/boyfriends may demand more of us.

But, please don't do what I did--don't expect to be perfect in those areas all the time because it will make you sick (emotionally, spiritually, and physically). Also, we working moms need to be "where we are, when we are" there. It's toxic to our mind-body-spirituality to be at work thinking we should be at home with the children and vice versa. Just living in the present moment decreases stress and thus helps tune the Hormone Symphony. If we are not living in the present moment, we are either living in the future which can bring dread or living in the past which can bring regret. Focus on the present—don't get bogged down in the future or the past. I must confess, however, that even with twelve years of practice as a working mom, I still struggle with this.

The best advice that I received lately was from my secretary who forwarded me one of those "great advice on the internet letters."

It was anonymous, but I believe very useful:
1. Pray.
2. Go to bed on time or early (the more sleep the better).
3. Get up on time so you can start the day unrushed.

4. Say "no" to projects that won't fit into your time schedule, or that will compromise your mental health.
5. Delegate tasks to capable others.
6. Simplify and unclutter your life.
7. Less is more. (Although one is often not enough, two is often too many.)
8. Allow extra time to do things and to get to places.
9. Pace yourself. Spread out big changes and difficult projects over time; don't lump the hard things all together.
10. Take one day at a time. Separate worries from concerns. If a situation is a concern, find out what God would have you do and let go of the anxiety. If you can't do anything about a situation, forget it.
11. Live within your budget and means; don't use credit cards for ordinary purchases.
12. Have backups; an extra car key in your wallet, an extra house key buried in the garden, extra stamps, etc.
13. K.M.S. (Keep Mouth Shut). This single piece of advice can prevent an enormous amount of trouble.
14. Do something for the Kid in You every day.
15. Carry a spiritually-enlightening book with you to read while waiting in line.
16. Get enough rest.
17. Eat right.
18. Get organized so everything has its place.
19. Listen to recorded audio while driving that can help improve your quality of life.
20. Write down thoughts and inspirations.
21. Every day, find time to be alone and have solitude.
22. Having problems? Talk to God on the spot. Try to nip small problems in the bud. Don't wait until it's time to go to bed to try and pray.
23. Make friends with Godly people.
24. Keep a record of favorite scriptures on hand.

25. Remember that the shortest bridge between despair and hope is often a good "Thank you, Jesus."
26. Laugh!
27. Laugh some more!
28. Take your work seriously, but not yourself at all.
29. Develop a forgiving attitude (most people are doing the best they can).
30. Be kind to unkind people (they probably need it the most).
31. Sit on your ego.
32. Talk less; listen more.
33. Slow down.
34. Remind yourself that you are not the general manager of the universe.
35. Every night before bed, think of one thing you're grateful for that you've never been grateful for before. God has a way of turning things around for you.

"If God is for us, who can be against us?" (Romans 8:31)

So, in summary, the take-home messages are:
Do what you love but maintain balance, don't rush (don't let time drive your adrenal glands), and develop an attitude of gratitude.

Tips for men

First, if you understand your woman, and that she just wants to be heard and not fixed, you are far better off than most other men, and she will love you for it.

Then if you love and respect her and her hormones, and listen to her as she expresses her feelings, you will have a much better relationship.

One day, I sat on a plane next to a 33-year-old man who was going to be married in three months. It was a long flight from Atlanta to Las Vegas and he found out what I do and he ended up asking me a lot of questions. It turns out that he met the most wonderful woman who was about 29 years old about two years ago. Last year, he proposed to her and she said yes. As they were older, they decided that they would try to have a honeymoon baby so she went off of her birth control pills about three months prior.

He said that since that time, she has become "a witch" right before her menstrual cycle. He describes her as tearful, moody, and downright vindictive. He's now considering calling off the wedding.

I gave him some basic advice to manage her PMS from a male perspective. I asked him to nod and listen and look sympathetic when she made comments about her abdominal bloating, her irritability, and her rings feeling tight. I told him to reassure her that she still looks great and to give her some Chasteberry herbs ("Vitex"), some Evening Primrose Oil and magnesium, and that she should see a doctor to consider progesterone cream.

He was so sincere, so confused, and so stressed about his fiancé, and this new personality he saw after she came off of her birth control pill, that I promised him that one day I would write an easy handbook for men, cartoons and all, entitled, *Is It Her, or Her Hormones? —a handbook for men who love their hormonal women.*

CASE STUDY: "The importance of love and forgiveness in care of the Conductor (and maybe some Oxytocin?)"

One day on vacation, I met a lady in South Florida who was just joyful, and bubbly. Her music was beautiful and I basked in it. A retired Exxon executive, I asked her what her secret was. She told me that in her previous job before retirement she was in the executive dog-eat-dog world and harbored a lot of stress, anxiety and resentment that was eating her alive. Then she discovered her secret to happiness.

I asked her to tell me. She looked me straight in the eye and said, "Angeli, it's very simple: all you have to remember is to **'Love everybody and forgive everybody, <u>EVERYTHING</u>.'**" She went on to explain that Jesus knew Judas was going to betray him and forgave Judas anyway. We have people in our lives—at work or at home or in our community—that rub us the wrong way or have hurt us, we need to forgive. Over the years since meeting her, I have tried out her hypothesis on myself and have shared it with my patients. I believe it is absolutely true.

Again, <u>lack for forgiveness is like drinking poison and hoping the other person dies</u>. It primarily hurts us and our Hormone Symphony.

I think that the one not often discussed and poorly understood factor in balancing the Hormone Symphony is <u>relationship</u> and that's why I am spending so much time on this. We do have clues in the medical literature—studies that suggest this with married men having longer lifespans than single men. Also, with newborn babies, the ones that are cuddled grow and develop better than the ones that are left in the cradle without enough human touch.

It's relationship, in my estimation, that can most positively or negatively affect our health and our Hormone Symphony.

I like that advice "love everybody and forgive everybody everything," because it is universal. You can be Christian, Buddhist, Hindu, Jewish, Muslim, agnostic or atheist and understand that axiom. I will tell you from a physiologic standpoint that harbored anger, resentment, and lack of forgiveness cause stress; stress drives the adrenal glands which increase cortisol/ DHEA and disrupts the rest of the symphony.

Oxytocin

There has been research on a hormone called "oxytocin," which is released when we hug each other. It's released at especially high levels as a new mom bonds with her baby, thus it's also called the "bonding hormone." We think that this directly combats cortisol. Some compounding pharmacists are selling this as a medication. I prefer the natural form of oxytocin; in fact, around my household, my boys are likely to hear "boys, mom needs some OXYTOCIN!" That means "can you come here and give mom a great, big hug?" For more on oxytocin, read *The Oxytocin Factor* by Kersitin Uvnas Moberg (Moberg, 2003).

MEN: ANDROPAUSE

CASE STUDY: "I feel like an old man"

Tim is a 43-year-old man who was athletic his whole life and who for the past six years has been in a high-stress marketing job, often traveling from his home in Florida to Chicago where he works during the week. He eats many meals out at restaurants and feels the drive to perform at work. He noted increasing abdominal girth, fatigue, loss of mental drive and loss of libido. He has to take a nap every afternoon despite six cups of coffee throughout the day. His work-outs are now lackluster. Everything is a chore. His labs have been progressing now with a high fasting blood sugar of 110mg/dL (goal under 90mg/dL), and his high LDL cholesterol at 190mg/dL (goal under 130mg/dL). His total testosterone is very low at 290ng/dL.

Case Analysis: Low Testosterone, metabolic syndrome, and adrenal fatigue

"I'm tired," "I'm getting fat," "I'm not recovering as well from my exercise," "I can't think clearly," "I don't think about sex," "I lost my edge"—these are all symptoms of low testosterone. So just replace testosterone and that's it?

I wish it were as easy as that; I would simply replace testosterone and my patients would be magically fixed. No, this is not the case, thus the utility of the Hormone Symphony model.

In discussing the Three Angles of Wellness (Box 1) with him, it turns out that he is not eating the right foods—mostly eating fast foods at the Atlanta airport. He is working out but hits the Chinese buffet line afterward. He has been weight training but not doing cardiopulmonary fitness training to burn abdominal fat, such as high intensity interval training (HIIT see Appendix A). He is driving his body on caffeine throughout the day so his sleep cycles were completely off at night. In addition, he has a lot of guilt about working in Chicago while his family lives in Florida (Box 2).

As for his family history, his mother had chronic diarrhea and died of undiagnosed dementia in her 70s, probably celiac disease. His father had died in his late 70s due to complications of cardiovascular disease and diabetes. He was a double amputee with wounds that wouldn't heal because of diabetes, and he had had a quadruple heart bypass.

Tim's treatment plan included stress management, adding high intensity interval training (HIIT) to his exercise regimen, going strictly gluten-free, cutting out simple carbohydrates that were driving up his insulin, and adding testosterone replacement by injection. He also included a protocol to decrease estradiol levels.

The results have been outstanding. Now, at age 46, he has his mental edge back, has lost 40 pounds, and has limitless energy and increased libido (I know because I am married to him). In fact, he is pursuing a career in action cinema thanks to his new physique. Balancing his Hormone Symphony has given him a second lease on life. He told me that the "tipping point" for him was back in 2007. I reviewed his labs he brought home from his doctor, looked at him and told him he was becoming like his father and that I would soon have to prepare to be an early widow. As I am not comfortable treating my own family, I have been in contact with his primary care doctor, his urologist, and his endocrinologist in advocating for him and the aggressive balancing of his Hormone Symphony.

The results? A picture is worth a thousand words.

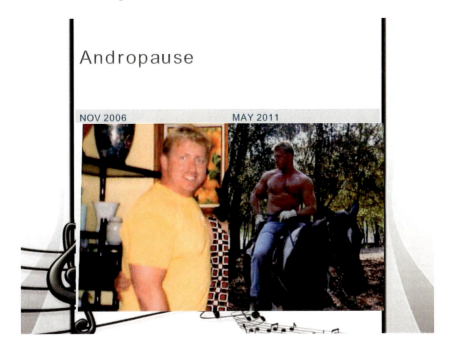

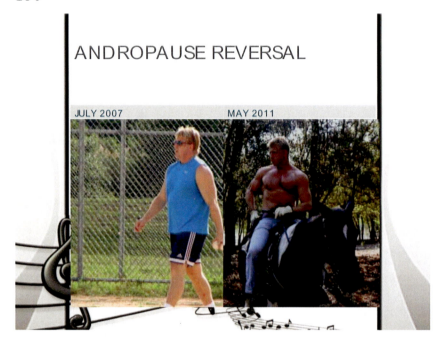

If you are a man, or if you have a man in your life that is concerned about the above—think "Hormone Symphony" (specifically, loss of testosterone). But remember, it's the whole symphony, not just a drug. Tim's amazing success was not due to only testosterone therapy, but hard work and nutrition as well. Tim finished his symphony.

More on this in **Part IV: Putting It All Together**.

From boys to men

Let's go back to children. If you have witnessed the transition from boys to men, think about the changes from "puberty." Mentally, you as a parent may remember as I do that when they would get hurt as a child, they would come to mommy for comfort, not caring who sees the tears in their eyes. When they were scared they would want to snuggle, and periods of intimidation from a big dog or an unknown such as skating or a new sport like football were very common. You may remember how your boys may have actually played with girls or even had a boy doll to nurture.

Then as the hormones changed (as evidenced by growth spurts, body odors, and acne), they started wanting to play with toy guns or the "shoot 'em up" video games, proclaimed "ew, yuck" in discussing girls, played rough and tumble and persistently poking at each other, and tears were suppressed as they expressed their fears, disappointments, and pains. That is, if they expressed them at all.

As full-blown adolescence occurred (which my boys have not arrived at yet, thank goodness), "risky behavior" and insatiable interest in girls occurs.

This is fairly well-known. What is not well-known or only recently known is the state of low testosterone—or **Andropause**, the opposite of male puberty. Now that pharmaceutical companies have spent money to patent new delivery systems (since natural bioidentical testosterone is not able to be patented), there tends to be much money to be made by these pharmaceutical companies if the general public starts to use these medications.

Thus, a hot topic has popped up in a public awareness campaign that was underwritten by a major pharmaceutical company to sell their testosterone, "Do you have Low T?" In my opinion, this has been the most effective campaign in bringing to men's attention the awareness that what they may have written off as normal male aging can be reduced or abated after all.

So although I have been replacing male hormones for years, I am grateful for this new campaign, which brings men into my office with this question in mind. Often they have already searched on the internet and have come in with clinical questionnaires filled out with the concern that they have low testosterone. This makes my job much easier.

Symptoms of low testosterone:
- Low energy, fast fatigue, slow energy return
- Getting fat (less lean muscle mass), especially belly fat!
- Poor recovery from exercise or less endurance – I had one patient who in his 40s quit playing basketball because his knees would hurt for two days after—with TRT (testosterone replacement therapy), this resolved; in addition, his borderline blood sugar and his high cholesterol improved markedly as his body fat lessened.
- Irritability, mood swings, oscillating ups/downs
- Erectile dysfunction/ low sexual libido
- Depression/Anxiety
- Lack of mental clarity, less decisiveness, short-term memory loss
- Loss of motivation, ambition, drive, "flatness"

In my office, I use an easy 10-point questionnaire called the ADAM score.
See: www.eje-online.org/content/151/3/355.full.pdf

A positive ADAM score has 81% sensitivity and 21% specificity for a low testosterone state. In other words, if you are a man with low testosterone, this questionnaire will be positive 81% of the time, but 21% of the time it will be positive for other conditions such as depression or drug side effects. (Tancredi, 2004)

Here are the questions:

The **Androgen Deficiency in Aging Males (ADAM)** questionnaire (answer Yes or No):
1. Do you have a decrease in libido (sex drive)?
2. Do you have a lack of energy?
3. Do you have a decrease in strength and/or endurance?
4. Have you lost height?
5. Have you noticed a decreased enjoyment of life'?
6. Are you sad and/or grumpy?
7. Are your erections less strong?
8. Have you noted a recent deterioration in your ability to play sport?
9. Are you falling asleep after dinner?
10. Has there been a recent deterioration in your work performance?

(Affirmative answers to questions 1 or 7, or to any three other questions indicate a positive result on the ADAM questionnaire.)

As for medication, I prefer the injectable testosterone because male hormones can transfer to my patients' loved ones from the topical creams and gels. Testosterone transfer to women and children can be dangerous. On more than one occasion, I have taken care of the wives of men on topical testosterone replacement and these women had high testosterone levels—they would come to me with complaints of acne, insomnia, irritability and weight gain. They had no need of testosterone at all; it caused a major imbalance in their Hormone Symphony. Also, I find a more even, steady state of hormones with injections. If my patient is needle phobic, I will use a testosterone patch.

Remember that replacing testosterone is for much more than just physique, strength, and preserving bone from deterioration (preventing osteoporosis) (Travison, 2006). The medical literature is pointing out now that testosterone is important in the preservation of memory and mental health (Atwood, 2005) and potentially in the prevention of Alzheimer's disease (Moffat, 2004) (Cherrier, 2005). It is very exciting, with our burgeoning epidemic of Type 2 diabetes, that there is much literature stating that optimizing testosterone is useful in the prevention of not only Alzheimer's, but metabolic syndrome as well—the precursor to Type 2 diabetes and other health problems (Muller, 2005).

This theory makes a lot of sense to me. It has been my observation that male patients with low testosterone present with depression, memory loss, and complaints of "having lost their edge." We now know that depression is considered a potential precursor to dementia. It is my observation that the lower their free testosterone, the worse their cognitive ability. Patients without enough testosterone feel like a wilted flower—they don't have enough water (hormones). The result: testosterone replacement therapy not only often cures erectile dysfunction (E.D.), but also mental status becomes more decisive, confident, alert, and more virile, <u>and memory improves</u>. In regards to diabetes prevention, this makes sense too—with less body fat and more lean muscle, insulin resistance goes down. Analogous to estrogen replacement therapy in women, there should be more research in testosterone replacement therapy as a possible preventative measure against Alzheimer's disease. <u>Hormone replacement may very well be the major modifiable epigenetic factor in the manifestation of Alzheimer's disease.</u>

Risks of testosterone replacement

Testosterone is not without its risks, unfortunately. The literature has some concerns about the potential for increased cardiovascular disease because of lowering of HDL (good cholesterol). However, with the data showing a reduction in metabolic syndrome with higher testosterone levels, this may balance out the risk.

Analogous to the concern about estrogen replacement therapy in breast cancer, there is concern about increased risk for prostate cancer with testosterone replacement therapy. The prostate cancer issue is currently debated, because there are many cases of prostate cancer where the men actually have low testosterone levels. This area is actively being researched (Rhoden, 2004).

But, I believe the theory that prostate cancer actually occurs because of an imbalance of estrogen to testosterone (at the level of the prostate gland tissue itself) will be found to be the primary contribution to prostate cancer. Stay tuned to this research.

Part III: B. Wind/Insulin (glucose) and metabolism

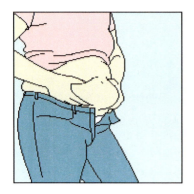

This is easy to recognize—just look at people's general shape. Become a people watcher at the mall. If the general shape of both men and women are apple shaped (waist larger than hips), think **metabolic syndrome**, and increased heart disease risk (which includes stroke risk) and increased risk for diabetes, not to mention poor energy handling. These people come to me with fatigue because their factories for energy handling are so inefficient.

We in America are in a perfect storm that is causing epidemic proportions of metabolic syndrome. Our lifestyle need for convenience has led us to have easy transportation with our multiple vehicles (which leaves us with an average of only 4,000 steps of walking per day as opposed to 10,000 steps per day for the rest of the world), the need for convenience foods like fast foods, pre-made dinners, eating out where the proportion per individual meal is often enough to feed a family of four, the "supersized meal," our machines that expend energy for us like our gas powered lawnmower as opposed to the push lawnmower, plus the mentality of "more is better", that larger proportions are better, plus our "have it done yesterday" mentality which drives our cortisol, which makes us crave salt and sugar and gain abdominal fat, which makes us insomniacs as we worry about the next day, which adulterates our appetite hormones leptin/ghrelin such that the ratios favor ghrelin which causes our appetite to increase (Spiegel, 2004), which makes us tired so we drive our adrenal glands with caffeine in the form of sodas, coffee, or energy drinks, which causes elevated cortisol levels for up to 48 hours and drives our appetite, which drives our food sources to make bread that is more doughy and smooth which has encouraged the U.S. food industry to genetically modify the foods to produce wheat that is more starchy so our bread is more soft and chewy which has probably driven up the rates of gluten sensitivity, which causes more inflammation which causes more fatigue which causes more hunger....

You get the picture. It's an unhealthy domino effect. If not, watch some food documentaries that are on Netflix™ that expose what is happening to our food sources in America. I suggest, if you are addicted to fast foods like my boys were, that you watch *Supersize Me*, a documentary about a man who was healthy and developed metabolic syndrome (pre- diabetes) and fatty liver after eating only McDonald's™ for just one month.

That movie, plus help from one of my patients, helped my boys make better food choices. A few years ago, I set up a trip to see a 70-year-old sweet patient of mine in the hospital post-operatively from a carotid endarterectomy (cleaning out the cholesterol plaques of the carotid artery) with my two boys. I called beforehand and told her to tell my boys that the blockages in her arteries were caused by foods that contained the same fat that is in McDonald's™. I can still see how they tentatively walked into her hospital room on rounds with me that day. As I took down the dressing on her neck to show them the stapled wounds, their eyes widened like they had seen Frankenstein! It cured them of their desire to eat another French fry again. It was one of those triumphant mommy moments. I am forever grateful to Mrs. Verna (who is now in heaven) for her generosity and spirit in helping me to help my boys kick their fast-food habit forever.

Another good movie is called *Forks Over Knives*, which features Dr. Esselstyne, a physician from the Cleveland Clinic, who wrote about reversing heart disease and whose vegan lifestyle is now followed by former President Bill Clinton. (Esselstyn, 2007)

I really believe that the key to reversing metabolic syndrome (and preventing diabetes) is dietary. It's all about taming the insulin by taming the glucose.

What is insulin? **Insulin** is a hormone produced by the pancreas in response to the amount of glucose (sugar and carbohydrates) that we eat. The impact of what we eat and how much the food is stimulating the pancreas to produce insulin is described as that food's **glycemic index**. When there is fiber in the food, it doesn't spike the insulin quite as high (which is good). This measurement of a food's impact on insulin (where it takes fiber into account) is called **glycemic load**. This difference is why you may have heard some diet books recommending you stay away from carrots (these are the ones that take into account only glycemic index, as carrots have high glycemic index but OK glycemic load because they have fiber).

In general, you do not have to pay too much attention to the difference. If you want to lose belly fat or put the lid on your metabolic syndrome if you are headed in that direction, from a nutritional standpoint, <u>make sure that you are eating foods with low glycemic index. If you happen to have a meal that has a high glycemic index food in it, balance it with a lot of fiber and/or protein.</u> This is why foods such as whole grain wheat breads are healthier than white breads, because their high fiber content blunts their high glycemic index.

For example, if you went to a Chinese restaurant and ate their typical meal of General Tsao's chicken, it would be laden with sugar in the sauce. If you do this, eat a lot of steamed broccoli and less white rice (which has a really high glycemic index, almost equal to that of table sugar). If you eat white bread, pasta, rice or potatoes you may as well have opened up your mouth and downed a scoop of granulated sugar!

It's not just Chinese food either, as we in America can take any ethnic food and make it unhealthy. For example, the true Italian Mediterranean diet is probably life preserving and helpful in reversing metabolic syndrome (Sacks, 2009). However, once it is "Americanized" with our larger portions and our genetically modified wheat pasta and pesticide-laden tomatoes, it becomes far less healthy.

The same is true with the American love affair with soda. Each 12-ounce can of Coca-Cola Classic™ has 10 teaspoons of granulated sugar! (Harvard School of Public Health) Genetically modified foods, processed carbohydrates, and sweetened drinks are wreaking havoc to our health as a nation. I advise all my patients to cut sugary sodas and drinks out of their diet. Not only is that much sugar unhealthy, the calories add up. Instead, drink water with lemon when you eat out at restaurants. If you must drink alcohol, do it sparingly and choose red wine (for its resveratrol).

Summary:
1. Metabolic syndrome, simply put, is a condition of abdominal fat accumulation which puts the individual at risk for heart attacks, strokes and diabetes (simplified definition, for official definition, see American Heart Association website).
2. The primary defect is excess insulin.
3. The primary maneuver to "tame" the insulin is to temper the sugar, so that the peaks, valleys, and waves of insulin following glucose are not as pronounced.
4. The dietary recommendation I give my patients is to <u>eat low glycemic index</u>, and to eat a lot of fiber.
5. Some references that explain this in detail:
   The South Beach Diet by Dr. Arthur Agatston
   Protein Power by Michael R. Eades
   Ultra-Metabolism by Dr. Mark Hyman
   The Idiot's Guide to Low Glycemic Index Weight Loss by Lucy Beale
   The Transitions™ brand weight loss program
   Ideal Protein™ brand weight loss program
   Weight Watchers™ low glycemic index subtype plan

Part III C: Percussion/Thyroid "The Rhythm Section"

I call this the Percussion or the Rhythm section because the thyroid gland acts as a "metabostat" to metabolism similar to how a thermostat controls temperature in a heating and air conditioning unit. It is known that the higher the levels of thyroid hormone, the faster the metabolism of your body. That's why in a pathological condition called Grave's disease where there is way too much thyroid hormone release, the symptoms are weight loss, tremor, and insomnia. It can even present as mania (rapid thinking and instability of mood); I had a patient present like this once.

The opposite of hyperthyroidism is hypothyroidism, or slow thyroid. That's why many of my patients who come to me with no medical knowledge at all tell me that they are overweight and they want their thyroid checked. Many of them are right. Many thyroids are running sub-optimally and so in turn, the patient's metabolism is suboptimal.

This is a touchy subject in traditional medicine and endocrinology. Most of us are taught that the thyroid is OK if the thyroid stimulating hormone (TSH) that comes from the part of the brain called the pituitary is < 3 µIU/mL. We are taught that if their TSH < 3 µIU/mL, the patient's symptoms of fatigue, hair loss, constipation, difficulty with losing weight, depression and constipation are not caused by the thyroid.

This is true most of the time but not all of the time. There are patients whose excessive stress (which releases excessive cortisol) causes the TSH from the pituitary gland to be low and so without further investigation, the patient can be written off as "euthryoid" or normal thyroid, and told he or she has those symptoms for genetic reasons or some other reason. I know because I used to be one of those physicians (about fifteen years ago when I first started my clinical practice, because I wasn't taught this in medical school or residency). Unfortunately, many of these patients find their way to these "weight loss centers" where they are given metabolism elevating medications such as phenteramine or phendrimethazine, which are simply resurrected forms of the infamous "Phen-fen" that was pulled off the market by the FDA in 1997 as it was found to cause heart valve problems and some lung problems.

In most of those cases, metabolism could simply be safely adjusted by fine-tuning the thyroid hormone or the Percussion section. Appropriate detailed thyroid testing in cases where I believe the patient may have hypothyroidism as the cause of symptoms like weight gain, constipation, depression, or memory loss would include not only the TSH, but the free T3, free T4, and reverse T3 (which goes up with too much stress). In medical school, we are taught reverse T3 increases when a patient is admitted to the intensive care unit with a disease which is overwhelmingly stressful in addition to the alarms and lack of sleep from the ICU setting itself; but I have found elevated reverse T3 in the community outpatient setting as well from the mere stress that our current U.S. society gives people as mentioned previously. I would also check anti-TPO antibodies, anti-thyroglobulin antibodies. (These are antibodies that target the thyroid gland, causing inflammation. More on this in the next section.)

In addition, I would be looking at the Conductor of the Hormone Symphony/ the adrenal glands—specifically the 4-point saliva test which most accurately reflects cortisol patterns throughout the day. If one draws an 8 a.m. blood cortisol, which is what we are taught to do in medical school, it would be elevated by the mere fact of the pain of the needle-stick itself. I believe 4-point saliva tests are more accurate (than the standard 8 a.m. blood test) in displaying real-time cortisol activity throughout the day. The salivary four point saliva tests have been validated in the U.S. medical literature by NASA studies and are still used to measure pilot stress levels.

Hashimoto's thyroiditis and acquired thyroid dysfunction

Hashimoto's thyroiditis is when the body attacks its own thyroid gland, or autoimmune thyroiditis, inflaming the tissue. It is overwhelmingly common in my practice, because I aggressively look for it. Basically, on tissue biopsy of the thyroid gland of people who have this condition, the thyroid tissue is unfortunately being attacked by their own lymphocytes. Lymphocytes are white blood cells involved in our immune system but somehow they got confused and started attacking the body. The best way to think about this is "friendly fire."

Lymphocytes were designed to survey and defend our bodies against viruses, cancer cells and certain bacteria such as tuberculosis. Somehow they got reprogrammed with autoimmune thyroid disease to fight the thyroid. One theory is that this confusion happened in the gut, at least in the case of gluten sensitivity.

In anatomy and histology, the basic sciences of medicine, I remember the pictures of the small bowel and how important it was in protecting against foreign invaders and absorbing nutrients. To sort this out, the small bowel is designed with cells that line up like a watertight fence so that only what should translocate or cross that barrier is allowed to cross like tollbooths. However, if there is allergy or food sensitivity, this fence becomes disrupted by a war that happens between the inflammatory cells and this protein or what, in the immune world, is called an "antigen." This war causes a lot of shrapnel and fallout, and a disruption in the enterocyte fence. When this happens, other proteins cross as well as the original protein that caused the problem. The immune system then becomes confused and starts mobilizing forces and the end result can be friendly fire, or autoimmunity.

Autoimmunity still has a lot of ongoing research behind it and we in medicine have a lot to learn, so the story is not completely clear. But for purposes of this discussion just remember:

Eating foods to which we have sensitivity → inflammation → breakdown in the integrity of the enterocyte wall → translocation of proteins → more inflammation → autoimmunity → illness.

This has been known for millennia in Chinese medicine and is described as "<u>leaky gut</u>."

In my clinical practice, when I have found Hashimoto's thyroiditis, I am looking at what caused the immune system to go awry.

[Hashimoto's thyroiditis often has the company of other autoimmune diseases such as vitiligo (loss of skin pigment) or alopecia (patches of hair loss) or multiple sclerosis (autoimmune disruption of the lining of nerves called the myelin sheath) or primary ovarian insufficiency commonly known as premature menopause, (Stazi AV, 2000) (Practice Committee of the American Society for Reproductive Medicine, 2004) or immune dysfunction, or autism or autistic spectrum disorders.]

With Hashimoto's thyroiditis, I have commonly found gluten sensitivity to be the cause. Actually, I am now in the habit for looking for gluten sensitivity in anyone who presents to my practice with an autoimmune process or a positive ANA (anti-nuclear antibody) blood test because if found, elimination of gluten can improve that person's health forever.

Gluten Sensitivity

There are two recent articles which have justified this aggressive approach to gluten sensitivity.

The first was published in a standard gastroenterological journal and acknowledged that there are ranges of gluten sensitivity. Like most things in medicine, it's not black and white, it's not that you have celiac disease or not. For most doctors, until recently, if the small bowel biopsy didn't show changes of the autoimmune damage from severe gluten sensitivity or celiac disease, then the patient didn't have gluten sensitivity at all.

This did not jive at all with what I was seeing clinically. I would see positive **celiac disease antibody titers** (or levels) in the blood, or the patient would have another autoimmune disease to make me think of gluten sensitivity, or the patient would come with a diagnosis of irritable bowel syndrome. (By the way, there was a study of only white women who were diagnosed with irritable bowel syndrome, and 30% had gluten sensitivity undiagnosed as the cause) (Green, 2007).

I would send these patients to the gastroenterologist specialist, who would do a small bowel biopsy through endoscopy, and the biopsy would come back normal. He/she would tell the patient that they don't have celiac disease, and the patient would therefore assume they could continue eating gluten—and they would eventually come back to me. And, as a primary care doctor, I would see them get sicker and sicker, rash after rash, cold after cold, allergy or asthma, stomach pains, work loss, and I would tell the patient to quit eating gluten but then they would retort how hard gluten-free eating is and how the stomach specialist said that they didn't have it anyway.

So now I provide them with these articles that say there is a spectrum of gluten sensitivity and that the diagnosis does not necessarily require a positive small bowel biopsy which is only obtained through endoscopy.

The first article is published in an academic professor's journal called *The American Journal of Medicine* last year from the Mucosal Biology Research and Center for Celiac Research at the University of Maryland in the fall of 2010 called "Celiac Disease Diagnosis: Simple Rules Are Better Than Complicated Algorithms."

It starts by saying: *"Celiac disease is the immune-mediated intolerance to dietary gluten, a protein contained in wheat, rye, and barley, affecting genetically predisposed individuals"* and makes a very bold statement: *"Celiac disease is the only treatable autoimmune disease, provided that a correct diagnosis is achieved and a strict, lifelong gluten-free diet is implemented."*

The article suggests that the diagnostic criteria be:

Diagnostic Criteria for Celiac Disease (at least 4 of 5 or 3 of 4 if the HLA Genotype is not performed)

1. Typical symptoms of celiac disease (examples of typical symptoms are chronic diarrhea, growth faltering [children] or weight loss [adults] and iron deficient anemia)
2. Positivity of serum celiac disease IgA class autoantibodies at high titer (Both IgA class TTG and EMA in IgA –sufficient or IgG class TTG and EMA in IgA – deficient subjects. The finding of IgG class anti-deaminated gliadin peptide adds evidence to the diagnosis)

3. HLA-DQ2 or HLA-DQ8 genotypes (but large studies show that 0.4% of celiac disease patients are both HLA-DQ2 and HLA-DQ8 negative)
4. Celiac enteropathy at small intestinal biopsy
5. Response to gluten-free diet (GFD); histological response in patients with sero-negative celiac disease or associated IgA deficiency (Catassi, 2010)

Basically, there is a spectrum of gluten sensitivity with celiac disease being at the center. But there does exist a <u>non-celiac gluten sensitivity</u> where the body still reacts immunologically, but to a lesser extent (Nejad, 2011). I use stool testing sometimes if the serum or blood testing is negative for celiac disease but I still suspect gluten sensitivity. You can order your own stool testing at Enterolab™ (see www.enterolab.com). Or you can ask your doctor to order you a blood test called ALCAT™ (see www.alcat.com).

Case Study: ALCAT™ testing for recalcitrant eczema

My sons were diagnosed with gluten sensitivity through ALCAT™ testing. The company that administers the ALCAT™ test, Cell Science Systems (CSS), has been in business for about 25 years. The book *Your Hidden Food Allergies are Making You Fat* (Deutsch and Rivera, 2002) explains about the procedures used for testing.

In general, it tests for delayed food sensitivities. ALCAT™ stands for Antigen Leukocyte Cellular Antibody Test. I usually order the ALCAT™ 200 Foods Sensitivity Test. Basically, a blood specimen is taken and the white blood cell component is isolated and divided up and placed in 200 individual tubes with 200 different foods. The results are analyzed at a microscopic level.

If there is no reaction at all, the food tested is considered safe and is listed in the green section of the test report. If there is some amount of reaction which is stimulating the immune system, it is labeled yellow (mild), moderate (orange), or severe (red) in progression based on the amount of reaction. The food that caused severe reactions should be eliminated forever (the red section of the report). The others can be rotated in the diet so eventually the sensitivity should go away.

You may only be aware of the classic acute food allergies like the boy who accidently eats a peanut and immediately has angioedema where he cannot breathe and his lips swell. He would need to be treated immediately with steroids, antihistamines and an epinephrine shot to stop the cascading abrupt immune reaction that can rapidly close off the airway and kill him. These are the so-called "IgE" mediated food allergies.

ALCAT™ tests for a different type of immune insult in which the time course is more insidious. The ALCAT is NOT an allergy or IgE test. It tests for food intolerances/sensitivities. It measures leukocyte (white blood cell) cellular reactivity in whole blood, which is a final common pathway of all mechanisms of food sensitivity or intolerance. For example, my younger son, Derek, as a toddler had chronic cough and severe skin eczema to the point where he would wake up with bloodied tissue under his fingernails. Eventually, the skin thickened up like an alligator's skin so the itching abated. No topical medication could correct this. Then at age 6, he had large enough tonsils that he was snoring and awakening at night from blockage of air caused by the size of the tonsils and his pediatrician referred him to a pediatric ENT surgeon to have his tonsils removed.

I did the ALCAT™ testing and found he had a severe reaction to beef and gluten. We eliminated these and all the other foods listed in the "red column" of the ALCAT™ test. It was hard for him at first because one of his favorite foods was the hamburger, and he loved apple pies. (At six years old, he even had his own apple pie company that was featured in our local paper, *The Gainesville Sun,* March 20, 2007 p. 4D.)

The good news was that eliminating foods ALCAT™ testing identified as causing him severe immune reactions resolved his rash, chronic cough and his tonsillar swelling. He no longer needed to have his tonsils removed surgically! The bad news was that he closed his apple pie company as he could not find a satisfactory gluten-free pie crust replacement.

Final notes on gluten sensitivity
My mother in law, Tim's mom, had a mysterious dementia in her 60's and died at 72 after she spent the last few years non-verbal in a nursing home under total care. Her symphony had stopped playing music. She had chronic diarrhea her whole life, especially after eating bread with their meals, and I suspect she had undiagnosed celiac disease which is now in the medical literature as a cause for dementia.

Tim also had gastroenterological problems and was diagnosed with gluten sensitivity with a stool Enterolab™ test showing antibodies. Our sons, Timothy Jr. and Derek, showed positive testing to gluten in the ALCAT™ tests.

All three have had clinical response to a gluten-free diet (GFD). To this day, whenever they have accidental gluten ingestion (in our house, we made up a term for this situation called "glutenized"), their symptoms return. We have to be very careful eating out.

Tim Sr. falls asleep within an hour and has stomach pain. Timothy, Jr. gets spacey and disoriented. Derek has stomach pain and a return of his dry cough within hours, and if he persists eating gluten, his skin rash returns as well.

We went to Rome for a week last Easter and threw caution to the wind and ate a lot of Italian pasta. With the ten miles per day of walking for sightseeing (Tim finds exercise helps him clear the inflammation when he is "glutenized", and this makes sense, as there are exercise physiology studies that have shown that exercise decreases inflammatory markers), only Derek had manifestations of his gluten sensitivity, and only on the flight home. He developed a facial rash as we boarded the return flight from Italy. By the time we made it home to Florida, the rash had worked its way down to his legs. He looked sunburned when he returned to class the next day. My doctor friends and I have discussed this and we believe that the genetically modified wheat we consume in the U.S. (that is banned in the European Union) gives us higher levels of gluten. That's why our bread is "fluffier" in Florida than Italy! I also think that's why the usual immediate reactions that Tim and the boys experience when "glutenized" did not occur on our trip to Italy. It seems the responses were dampened there.

In Chinese medicine, one basic principle is that if there is an adverse outcome to a food, then avoid it. It's like recommending that someone not go back to touch a hot stove if he/she was burned touching it in the first place. Food sensitivities such as gluten do indeed give a low level of fire, or inflammation, when ingested. As I discussed in the first chapter, inflammation and oxidation are the two main ways of accelerating the aging of tissues. Elimination of foods and substances that have a bad outcome seems logical, and I recommend my patients do so regardless of the results of testing.

However, if you are suspecting after reading this that you may have gluten sensitivity spectrum-related inflammation, which can cause the classic manifestations of stomach pains, diarrhea, abnormal liver function studies, rashes, dementia, fatigue or other auto-immune disease, I would strongly suggest you discuss this with your physician and have testing done.

If you do not have the resources for testing, I believe it is also reasonable to take the Chinese medicine approach. <u>Eliminate gluten completely</u> for 8 to 12 weeks and see if your symptoms go away. If it does go away, this is called a clinical response to a gluten-free diet and is one of the new criteria in the diagnosis of celiac disease. The only difficulty that I have seen, as in my own family, is that once you have eliminated gluten and feel better, the sensitivity of testing for celiac disease as opposed to the lesser form of gluten sensitivity is difficult. In other words, while on a gluten-free diet, the inflammation can go down so much that the blood and tissue criteria for diagnosis go away, and tests would not find anything. Essentially, the patient went into remission from the disease. It's really hard to tell a patient "OK, now that you feel better, go back to eating gluten and feeling badly so I can make a definitive diagnosis of your celiac disease/ gluten sensitivity." There is a lot of research emerging right now in the medical literature on the topic of gluten intolerance.

For more information on this topic, which I believe is an understated but major public health problem, please look at the internet resources. The Celiac Disease Foundation's website (<u>www.celiac.org</u>) is updated and useful. Also there are gluten intolerance support groups in most areas and many websites that blog on recipes and strategies to maintaining a gluten-free lifestyle. Just remember a basic principle, if you are gluten sensitive to any extent, don't "stoke the fire" or cause smoldering inflammation by "just eating *one* cookie," for example. You can't make exceptions on the GFD. In other words, try to stay 100% gluten free as best that you can because elimination of any cause of inflammation in your body is a basic principle to playing beautiful music with your Hormone Symphony.

Part III D. Brass Section/Vitamin D

This is the "structure" of the Hormone Symphony. As brass is hard, I think of the Brass section as the structure behind the Hormone Symphony. Without structure, it doesn't matter how well the other parts of the Hormone Symphony play. If one's bones are weak, then one cannot function or play well at any age. Literally, with weak bones or osteoporosis, I ban skiing, contact sports or roller-blading, and I aggressively screen for fall-risks.

Within the past few years, Vitamin D was promoted to a hormone because it has effects on practically every cell in the body like other hormones. I explain to my patients that it was the opposite of what happened to Pluto, the planet that was demoted to a rock based on criteria. Vitamin D was promoted from vitamin to hormone because in addition to its well-known effect on bone health, it affects the brain and acts like an anti-depressant, it supports cell-mediated immunity, and in some studies it prevents colon and breast cancer. In other words, it acts more like a hormone affecting every cell in the body.

The actual level optimal level of 25-hydroxy Vitamin D has been debated, but in general, I aim for a level of around 60 ng/mL (Holick, 2007).

CASE STUDY: "Bone health and early menopause"

I met a 41-year-old woman who came in because she had trouble with her memory and was tired all the time. She had been diagnosed with primary ovarian insufficiency (her ovaries failed at age 21). This was discovered when her menstruations stopped abruptly. Due to poor medical access and "not wanting to deal with it," she had only been on female hormone replacement therapy for about 2 of the past 21 years. The standard recommendation would have been to give her estrogen replacement at least to keep her bones healthy, not to mention her skin and mind and other tissues healthy at least until age 51 when menopause usually occurs (Nelson, 2009).

She brought old blood work from 1998, at age 28, that included FSH that was high (signaling her brain trying to wake up her ovaries), a prolactin level that was normal (meaning she did not have a pituitary tumor causing her to stop her menstruations), a TSH at 4.31 µIU/mL, positive anti–thyroxperoxidase (anti-TPO was positive consistent with Hashimoto's thyroiditis), and an ANA (anti-nuclear antibody) that was negative (which would argue against lupus and used as a general screen for autoimmunity). She had negative (zero) celiac disease antibody titers in the blood.

However, she presents a history that since that time, she has figured out that whenever she eats gluten she feels tired, with an upset stomach, so she started avoiding it on her own.

She was lost to medical follow-up until 2010, at age 40, when she saw a friend who is a physician as she was tired and she had labs that showed:

Parathyroid hormone was normal, 25-hydroxy Vitamin D was 37 ng/mL (goal is about 60 ng/mL), urinary n-telopeptide was normal showing she was not urinating out bone metabolites (a good sign), DEXA bone density showed progression of lumbar or

back osteopenia and she had the bones of a 50-year-old woman with a lumbar T score of negative 2.8 (it was negative 2.5 at age 30, so progression had occurred) [BRASS section].
TSH was high at 14 µIU/mL, and free T4 was low at 0.9 µIU/mL, showing slow thyroid from the autoimmune thyroid disorder, Hashimoto's thyroiditis [PERCUSSION section].

I met her just recently at age 41, and upon physical exam, she looked much older than 41, with a facial wrinkle pattern more consistent with 50. She also had glabellar wrinkles between the eyebrows which she said were even treated with Botox™ and "marionette lines" around her mouth.

Recent studies have associated facial wrinkles (especially glabellar wrinkles) with bone health, as both skin and bone have to do with structure. Dr. Ruth Freeman, Principal Investigator of a study at Yale Medical School, explained that the skin and the skeleton have the same collagen. So when the collagen breaks down and you lose bone density, the collagen in the skin (which we can openly see) also breaks down causing visible wrinkles and other changes in the skin thickness. The study was presented at the 2011 annual meeting of the American Society of Endocrinology in Boston.

Case Commentary

As I have just met this patient, I explained to her that her efforts in the care of her Conductor have paid dividends. I instructed her to continue her exercise, organic eating and primarily non-meat diet (Box 1). Although she was initially mourning the loss of her fertility years ago, she is now happy at home, married and nurturing her 9-year-old step-daughter (Box 2). In regards to the sections of her Hormone Symphony, I advised her that we should be aggressive at replacing her hormones (STRINGS section, sex hormones), and it may not only be estrogen, it will probably be testosterone and progesterone as well. I ordered saliva testing and serum hormone testing.

I believe that her fatigue, memory loss, lack of libido, and premature wrinkling and osteopenia has to do primarily with estrogen but also has contribution from low testosterone and progesterone, which are also made in the ovaries.

I told her that though her celiac titers were negative, as she does have anti-TPO antibodies and hypothyroidism indicating Hashimoto's thyroiditis, [Percussion section, thyroid], and symptomatic relief of stomach irritation with avoidance of bread, she was probably gluten sensitive. She may very well have non-celiac gluten sensitivity and her premature ovarian insufficiency may be caused by an autoimmune process. I told her that I would be doing secondary testing for gluten sensitivity, including HLA DQ-2 and HLA DQ-8 testing. In addition, I would be continuing to replace her thyroid hormone, as she is fatigued.

For her osteopenia (early stages of osteoporosis), I explained that she needs at least 1500 mg of usable calcium and to continue her resistance training. At this point, the combination of weight-bearing exercise, increasing her calcium intake, optimizing her Vitamin D, and the addition of hormone replacement would be the preferred treatment plan. I would recheck a bone density in twelve months instead of the usual 24 months (BRASS section).

If her HLADQ-2 or HLADQ-8 testing came back positive, I would have enough evidence that perhaps it was gluten sensitivity that incited the friendly fire against both her thyroid and her ovaries, and I would advise a strict gluten-free diet for at least 2-3 months. During this time, though chances are slight because it has been over twenty years since her last menstruation, her ovaries may wake up and start functioning again. A return of a menstrual period and fertility would signal the return of healthy ovaries, and this has been reported in the literature. (Stazi, 2000).

We have a lot of opportunities to fine-tune her Hormone Symphony.

PART IV: Putting It All Together

Putting it all together

"Feed your dreams and your doubts will starve themselves to death".
        --Unknown

I am going to use my husband Tim's case (see Andropause Section IIIA to refresh your memory) as a demonstration of how to put it all together. Knowing him since I was 17 years old, it was scary to see his health rapidly decline about five years ago. He was just not himself and I knew a lot of it was due to his stressful marketing job that required frequent travel away from home, often to Chicago. I was here in Florida with our two young boys, and we would pray every night that "daddy would come home."

It then happened a few summers ago that his particular position was terminated, allowing Tim to be home and have balance in his life. This was the answer to our prayers.

He had already been starting to make progress with his Hormone Symphony when he was changed to injectable testosterone and started to exercise, but it was not until this major lifestyle change – the change from the high-stressed, high-powered vocation, to one of local responsibility that kept him home at night, that really made a positive change in his health and quality of life.

But for the sake of understanding how to plot a symphony, let's use Tim's experience and start from the beginning.

In (Box 1) of the Advanced Hormone Symphony:
Tim improved when he no longer felt the guilt of not seeing the boys during the week. (He missed an entire season of basketball where our younger son, Derek, was the star player.)

He started eating less of the SAD diet (see previous discussion) and was making changes for salads and chicken breasts without the dressing, even in the Atlanta airport. He began to carry healthy snacks like protein bars and nuts. He stayed hydrated with 2 liters of water per day and gave up on the soda and excessive caffeine that was driving his adrenal glands. I encouraged him to quit microwaving food in plastics and quit drinking out of plastic water bottles. This is known to release bisphenol A, which is an estrogen-like compound. He was already struggling with his abdominal fat which was converting his testosterone to estrogen, so he needed to stay away from these chemical "endocrine disruptors" (Diamante-Kandarakis, 2009). There is currently active research in this area with a negative study published looking at the association between bisphenol A and Type 2 diabetes in China (Bi, 2011). I'm glad there is active research in this area.

In addition, I introduced Tim to HIIT (high intensity interval training) for cardiopulmonary fitness. This was to drive his metabolism and burn belly fat at rest. This works great for my busy executives because a full program is only 16 minutes four days per week (see Appendix A).

Also, he totally cut out gluten (his stool studies came back positive for antibodies against tissue transglutaminase [anti-TTG] through Enterolab™, and his chronic diarrhea resolved). I encouraged him to get 20 minutes of sun per day and sleep without his cell phone and digital alarm clock and laptop next to him like he used to (eliminating electromagnetic radiation in the night environment). In addition, he took melatonin and L-theanine supplements to go into deep sleep at night. His naps were encouraged unless it disrupted night sleep (this is called "sleep hygiene"). He also began Krav Maga martial arts and running the stadiums with a weighted vest at the University of Florida, (the "Swamp"), which became both his exercise and meditative time. In addition, he did short bursts of high intensity weight training five times per week and I increased his protein intake while healing his gut.

In (Box 2), Tim has resolved the conflict between career advancement and spending time with his family.
In the symphony sections itself, his STRINGS section needed the most tuning, as he had low testosterone at 290 ng/dL.

I suspect (though not tested specifically), with Tim's gluten sensitivity, he probably had antibodies working against his testicles which caused "primary gonadal failure" at a young age. His testosterone level at age 42 should not have been less than 300 ng/dL. Even the most conservative endocrine societies would say this is too low. His level was <u>less than half</u> of the average for his age.

In fact, observational studies have shown that testosterone does naturally decline with age. A male patient should have at least the average testosterone level for his age group. However, I agree with many Age Management Medicine specialists to replace testosterone up to the 35-year-old level, the peak of health.

Average Testosterone Levels by Age in Men

Measurements in Conventional Units **(ng/dl)**, SHBG in (nmol/L)

Age	Number of Subjects	Total Test	Stand. Dev.	Free Test	Stand. Dev.	SHBG	Stand. Dev.
25-34	45	617	170	12.3	2.8	35.5	8.8
35-44	22	668	212	10.3	1.2	40.1	7.9
45-54	23	606	213	9.1	2.2	44.6	8.2
55-64	43	562	195	8.3	2.1	45.5	8.8
65-74	47	524	197	6.9	2.3	48.7	14.2
75-84	48	471	169	6.0	2.3	51.0	22.7
85-100	21	376	134	5.4	2.3	65.9	22.8

Vermeulen, A. (1996). *Declining Androgens with Age: An Overview.*

As you can see from the chart, Tim's testosterone levels were normal for someone over 80 years old, not 42. I encouraged his primary doctor and endocrinologist to drive his testosterone levels to 35-year-old levels, the known peak of health (for more details, see Appendix B).

Doing this has also resolved his WIND section/Metabolism section with complete remission of his metabolic syndrome. His thyroid and Vitamin D were checked and were optimal already.

The results have been tremendous. As a woman, I think Tim looks fabulous. He is even working on a career as an action hero in the world of cinema and film (see the story in his home town paper in upstate New York, http://pressrepublican.com/0100_news/x1756377831/Clintonville-native-has-the-looks-for-German-sci-fi-thriller).

I am glad his memory has returned and his energy is boundless. He's optimistic and his libido is unbridled, like he was in his early 30s. His symphony was so "off" five years ago; we were more like brother and sister than husband and wife.

As a physician, I am relieved that he has reversed his metabolic syndrome. He is down to 10% body fat, his LDL cholesterol is down from 190mg/dL (dangerously high) to 120 mg/dL without statin medications that are so prevalent today, and his hemoglobin A1C went from 5.9 mmol/mol down to an optimal 4.9 mmol/mol. (Diabetes is diagnosed when the hemoglobin A1C is greater than 6.5 mmol/mol, and the lower the better, with optimal being 5.2 mmol/mol or less.)

He is far from diabetes now, and having known his father who died of complications of diabetes in a very slow fashion, first with cardiovascular disease diagnosed in his 60s, then a double amputation after peripheral vascular disease in his 70s I am extremely grateful. And knowing his mother, who all her life had chronic diarrhea and died of an undiagnosed dementia which I suspect was undiagnosed celiac disease, it's nice to know that Tim will be around for a lot longer now for me and the boys who adore him so much.

Tim's Regimen

Tim is now playing beautiful music with his finely-tuned Hormone Symphony. He has graciously provided the exercise and nutrition regimen he has developed that has given him such amazing results (Box 1). Keep in mind that in Age Management Medicine, it is the <u>whole symphony</u> that matters. Now is the time to review the inside back cover of this book. I have many patients on injectable testosterone who have not changed anything else in their symphony and have had little to no improvement at all.

Tim Akey's Exercise Training Method

<u>Daily Supplement Protocol</u> includes:
- CoQ-10
- Vitamin D3
- Conjugated linoleic acid
- Omega-3 fatty acids
- L-carnitine
- Diindolmethane (DIM)
- Saw palmetto
- Zinc glycinate
- general multivitamin

<u>Pre-workout elixir:</u>

- L- carnitine
- D-ribose
- Alpha lipoic acid
- CoQ-10
- Creatine
- Mighty Maca™ greens drink
- Arginine
- Resveratrol
- and "eat an apple on the way to gym to stabilize the blood sugar"

<u>Training Regimen:</u>

- *Stadium runs (going up and down steps) with a 40lb. weighted vest 2-3X/week. Goal of at least 600 calories burned. [HIIT cardiovascular exercise strengthens the heart and lungs (see Appendix A). When Tim finishes his exercise at the stadium, I can smell the ketones on his breath for hours, which means his body is actively burning fat.]*

- *Strap on a Polar™ f4 heart rate monitor. Use the Karvonen™ formula calculation to assess target heart rate and achieve maximum efficiency.*
- *Krav Maga martial arts 2x/week*
- *Weight training: 5 days/week.*
- *Resistance training style: rapid succession—multiple sets on same body part. This increases intensity and cuts down on training time.*

<u>Post-training:</u>

- *20 gram whey protein shake for muscle repair (to be taken within 30 minutes of finishing exercise)*
- *A balanced, non-sugary electrolyte solution*

Commentary

Tim's exercise and nutraceutical program is unique because he's training for a potential movie role. It's a good idea to get the approval of your doctor before beginning any exercise program. I would encourage middle-aged male patients to have a cardiopulmonary fitness assessment before engaging in any training, especially one as rigorous as Tim's. Also, hiring a personal trainer to avoid injury is a good investment.

Remember, Tim worked up to this level of fitness. My exercise prescription outlined in the HIIT diagram (Appendix A) provides a satisfactory training program from beginners ("couch potatoes"), to intermediate level (like me), to advanced level training. The most important thing you can do is to get up and start moving. Choosing to exercise is always harder than the actual exercise itself!

140

Part V: Plot Your Own Hormone Symphony

Plot Your Own Hormone Symphony

"I must finish [writing this letter] now, because I've got to write at breakneck speed—everything's composed—but not written yet."
      --Wolfgang Amadeus Mozart

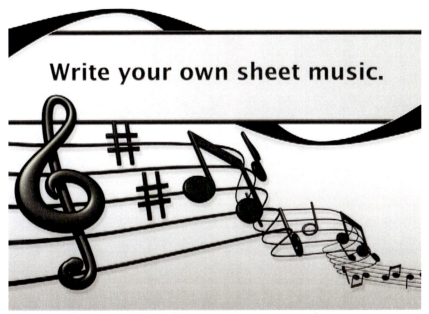

Now, reader, you are ready to write your own sheet music.

You intuitively know what it will take to make beautiful music with your Hormone Symphony. The music is inside of you. Now let's spend a few minutes and plot your Hormone Symphony, so you will have a wellness road map, the sheet music, to direct you in fine-tuning your Hormone Symphony.

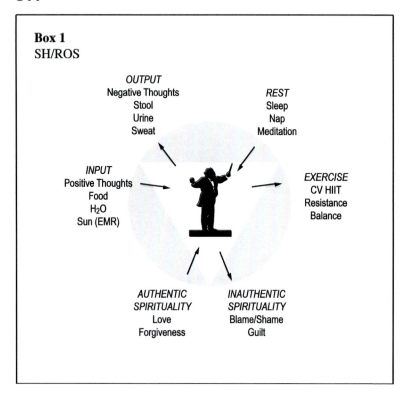

Box 1: Angle 1
INPUTS:
1. Am I feeding my mind with thoughts of gratitude? Is my "self-talk" affirming and life-sustaining?
2. Am I eating whole foods that are organic, non-processed, and non-hormonal, with the optimal 9 – 11 fruits and vegetables servings per day? Am I eating wild fish high in omega 3 fatty acids?
3. Am I drinking at least 2 Liters of filtered water daily?
4. Am I getting 20 minutes of non-peak sunshine per day which helps my Vitamin D and mood?

OUTPUTS:
1. Am I frequently purging negative thoughts and refusing to dwell on the past? If I am not living in the present, I am living in the past (regret) or the future (dread).
2. Do I have at least one to two good bowel movements per day?
3. Is my urine clear? Am I drinking enough water?
4. Do I sweat daily for detoxification?

Angle 2
REST:
1. Do I get at least 6-8 hours of uninterrupted sleep at night? If not, what is impeding this? Do I drink too much caffeine in the afternoon? Do I exercise too close to bedtime? Do I eat 2 hours before bedtime? Does my partner say that I snore? Do I wake up tired and want to nap in the daytime? Could I have sleep apnea? Do I have appropriate sleep hygiene? Do I keep the room dark at night? Do I keep all electronics out of my bedroom including the digital alarm clock, the laptop, and the television? Do I sleep in silence? (If you cannot sleep in total silence, buy an air filter. It will keep background noise steady so that you will not be subconsciously processing the sound, and it will also clean the air.)
2. Do I need a nap between 3 and 5 p.m.? If so, does this interrupt my deep sleep at night (if this does interrupt deep sleep, please skip the nap).
3. Do I meditate, pray, or do relaxation exercises daily?

EXERCISE:
1. Do I engage in cardiovascular exercise daily? Do I walk the minimum activity requirement of 10,000 steps daily (about 5 miles)? Do I have abdominal fat to burn and if so, am I doing high-intensity- interval training at least 4 days per week? (see Appendix A)
2. Do I do any resistance training to strengthen my muscles and bones? This could be pushups, sit-ups and pull ups, this could be Pilates™, strength training (please use a personal trainer), or plyometric exercises (see www.bodyrock.tv for a great home workout).
3. Do I do any balance training? This could be Tai Chi, yoga, dancing or balance classes.

Angle 3

1. Authentic Spirituality
Does my spirituality lead me to "love everyone and forgive everybody everything"? Do I practice the principles of my spirituality daily? Do I pray?
2. Inauthentic Spirituality
Does my spirituality lead me to feeling blame, shame, or guilt? If so, what needs to change here?
** A helpful book in this area that distinguishes the two and helps in areas of forgiveness is called *The Shack* by William Paul Young (2008).

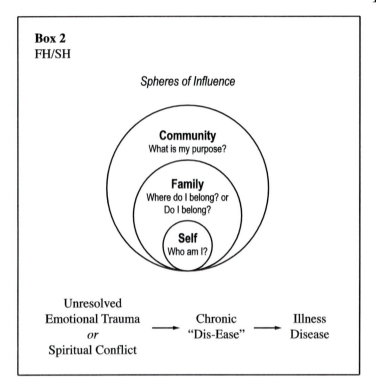

Box 2:

1. <u>Self</u>
   Who am I? Do I have a positive self-image? Do I love myself? Am I grateful for the experiences both difficult and easy that have brought me to the place I am now? Can I let go of any regret, resentment, or anger I have against someone or some event that did me harm in the past? The pitfall to having a good self-esteem is having childhood wounds that are not addressed.

2. <u>Family</u>
   Where do I belong? Am I happy in my current "home"? Am I able to be completely intimate with someone in my life? Am I able to share with this

person who I am without my mask(s) and feel accepted and loved unconditionally? Do I feel like I am trying to prove myself in my family of origin? Have I moved from adolescence to adulthood with my parents? Have I forgiven my mom/dad for not being perfect? Do I trust my family to be there for me? The pitfall here is unresolved emotional trauma. Was there an event in my childhood that was so traumatic that it has been suppressed?

3. <u>Community</u>
   What is my purpose in life? Do I feel that I am contributing to society? Do I feel like I wake up with a purpose in life? Who am I serving? Why am I serving them? The pitfall here is an incomplete understanding of worth.

With the current economy and unemployment reaching 10%, many of my patients have incorrectly put their entire worth as a person in their job or material security. When they become unemployed, their entire universe collapses. The key here is to make sure they know that they are valuable as a person regardless of their employment or their material things.

I have also found that many of my patients "crash" physically or emotionally when there is active movement in 2 or 3 Spheres of Influence. They come in with acute anxiety or depression or incapacitating fatigue. For example:
- I have seen a patient lose his job (Self and Community Sphere) and learn his son was diagnosed with cancer (Family sphere), which resulted in acute, incapacitating anxiety.
- I have seen a patient that finally felt free to be his authentic self after the death of his Controller-mask mother (Self Sphere). Though he now had freedom, he

also missed his mother; this conflict of positive and negative caused major depression (Family sphere).

Box 3:

1. <u>Acute Illness</u>
   Do I have anything troubling me right now? Am I short of breath? Do I have chest pain? Do I have abdominal pain? Do I have back pain? Are my bowels irregular?
2. <u>Chronic Illness</u>
   Do I have diabetes? Heart disease? Cancer? If so, how are these managed? Are they in good control or remission?
3. <u>Past Surgical History</u>
   Do any of my previous surgeries affect me today? Do I have scar pain or chronic pain from any of my surgeries?
4. <u>Past Trauma History</u>
   Is there any trauma that is still affecting me today?
   Physical traumas - Have I had a concussion? Have I been in a car accident? Have I broken a limb?

Box 3
Current Illness/PMH/PSH

70% of primary care complaints here

Acute Illness

Chronic Disease

Past Surgical History

Past Trauma History (physical or emotional)

Emotional traumas - Have I been involved in a war in any way? Have I been the victim of a crime? Am I the child of an alcoholic? Have I ever been emotionally/sexually abused? Have I ever been forced to act in an intimate way without my consent? Have I been abused by my parent/spouse/friend/boyfriend/girlfriend/other?

The above Boxes (Box 1, 2, and 3) are very useful in evaluating the state of you, the Conductor.

Know that it is true—I cannot separate the body from the mind from the spirit.

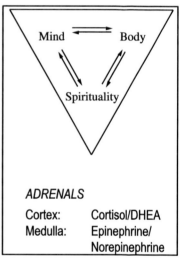

Somewhere the net effect is driving the adrenal glands. Reaction to stress is completely individual and completely personal; essentially the metaphorical "big, black box". I tried to dissect it well but I think the net effect is only an approximation of understanding the Conductor. The Chinese call it the "Chi", which means "energy life force". I like this description better, it's more general and less confining.

You have the ability to control how your body reacts to stress to a great degree. In other words, you, the Conductor, hold the baton. The baton to me represents the release of stress hormones which essentially drives the entire Hormone Symphony.

Acute stress is like what happens when being chased by an alligator. It releases epinephrine and norepinephrine from the adrenal glands' center, called the medulla. These are also known as catecholamines. It allows the body to quickly ramp up its metabolism to get out of an acutely dangerous situation.

Chronic stress is more insidious and releases cortisol/DHEA from the outer parts of the adrenal glands called the cortex. These, as mentioned above, occur when the body is stressed and it hyper-functions (remember, "hyperadrenia"), but eventually burn-out occurs—"hypoadrenia" or more casually called "adrenal fatigue."

The reasons why I extensively reviewed the masks we all wear are because it has everything to do with our relationships with others and how we perceive our place in the world. Like everything else in our bodies, there is a genetic component to our personality types but much can be modulated through our own internal work. I would encourage you to do the internal work to balance your CONDUCTOR, so you can balance your Hormone Symphony and make beautiful music.

Now, go to the HORMONE SYMPHONY on the foldout last page and enter in slot 1 one major change you will start doing today from Box 1. Enter in slot 2 an area that needs to be healed from Box 2. Enter in slot 3 an illness/condition that needs to be addressed with your doctor.

On to the Sections of the Symphony

Strings Section/ Sex Hormones
(Estrogen/Progesterone/Testosterone)

For women: (rate 1 for never and 5 for always)
1. Am I having difficulty concentrating and remembering?
2. Am I having hot flashes and /or night sweats?
3. Lack of sexual desire?
4. Feeling anxious?
5. Mood swings?
6. Feeling depressed, sad or unhappy?
7. Difficulties with sleep?
8. Irritability or nervousness?
9. Heart palpitations?
10. Changes in length of my menstrual cycle?
11. Changes in the amount of menstrual bleeding?
12. Breast tenderness?
13. Bloating or fluid retention?
14. Weight gain?
15. Vaginal dryness?

If you score between 45 and 75, this indicates strong likelihood of hormone imbalance. However, pay attention to where you may have scored high on one, two, or three questions. This may also indicate a hormone imbalance. (See **www.womeninbalance.org** for more details.)

For men:
The Androgen Deficiency in Aging Males (ADAM) questionnaire (answer Yes or No):
1. Do you have a decrease in libido (sex drive)?
2. Do you have a lack of energy?
3. Do you have a decrease in strength and/or endurance?
4. Have you lost height?
5. Have you noticed a decreased enjoyment of life?
6. Are you sad and/or grumpy?
7. Are your erections less strong?
8. Have you noted a recent deterioration in your ability to play sports?
9. Are you falling asleep after dinner?
10. Has there been a recent deterioration in your work performance?

Affirmative answers to questions 1 or 7, or to any three other questions provide a positive result on the ADAM questionnaire.

If your screen was positive, mark the Strings section for further investigation with your physician.

Wind/Metabolism (Insulin/ Glucose) Section
1. If I am a woman, is my waist greater than 35 inches* (measured through both anterior hip bones and through the belly button)?
2. If I am a man, is my waist greater than 40 inches*?
3. Do I have sugar cravings?
4. If I don't eat for two to three hours, do I get irritable, confused or angry?
5. Am I tired easily?
6. Do I have a family history for diabetes or heart disease?
7. (Female) Did I have diabetes during pregnancy?
*Caucasian measurements. These recommendations vary by race.

If any of these questions are positive, please have laboratory testing with your physician who will look for markers of insulin resistance such as high fasting sugar, high fasting insulin, high fasting triglycerides, and high markers of inflammation like C – reactive protein. In addition, an "HgbA1C" measurement which represents the average of blood sugar during the previous 90 days would be helpful.

Percussion Section/Thyroid (TSH/ Free T3/ Free T4)
1. Do I exercise and eat right and am still not able to lose weight or fat?
2. Am I depressed or foggy-brained?
3. Do I feel cold when everyone else is hot?
4. Is my morning body temperature below 97.8 F orally?
5. Am I constipated?
6. Am I losing hair?
7. Do I have high cholesterol?
8. Am I sluggish?
9. Does my skin feel doughy? Do I look doughy (bags under my eyes, rings tight?)
10. Do I have bumps or nodules on my thyroid?

If any of these questions are positive, please have your doctor order further blood work that should include detailed thyroid tests [TSH, Free T3, Free T4, anti – thyroperoxidase antibodies (anti-TPO antibodies), and if under a great deal of stress, order a reverse T3 (rT3)].

Brass Section/ Vitamin D
1. Have I had any fractures?
2. Do I get at least 20 minutes on non-peak sun exposure daily?
3. Does mom or dad have osteoporosis?
4. Do I take at least 1500 mg of calcium in my diet daily?

5. Am I on medications that make my bones weak like steroids for autoimmune disease or seizure medications? Do I have thyroid disease, or any inflammatory disease such as rheumatoid arthritis or lupus or ulcerative colitis that can make by bones weak?

If any of the above are positive, or even if not, with the current prevalence of low Vitamin D (30 to 50% of Americans by some estimates), please have your Vitamin D checked in the form of 25-hydroxy Vitamin D. Your doctor may also consider ordering a bone density scan ("DEXA" scan).

Conclusion

So there you have it. You have had your first run at understanding you, the Conductor, and understanding the hormone hierarchy where if the Conductor is not right (no matter if each part of the Hormone Symphony is tuned), you do not feel right. So the first order of business is to tune the Conductor. You control the tempo of the baton which moves the Hormone Symphony. Think of the baton as releasing substances from the adrenal glands that control the rest of the symphony. With acute stress, these are catecholamines which work in seconds to minutes. With chronic stress, DHEA and cortisol are released—these work in minutes to days to years, but eventually "burn-out."

Review the inside back cover of the book for the final time. Do you see how the Conductor stands on Box 1, 2 and 3? Think of these as the stage on which the Conductor stands. These are foundational. It's very important to care for the Conductor in ways outlined in Box 1, to understand the Conductor with questions in Box 2, and to address illnesses and traumas as outlined in Box 3.

Then and only then are you ready to balance the rest of the Hormone Symphony. Although, in my practice I will attempt to do all of them simultaneously, the best results occur when the Conductor is healthy first and then I work with the individual hormone sections. This approach will fine-tune your Hormone Symphony.

I hope this guide has helped you. For more information on this and other topics, please see my website:
www.agelessmedicalsolutions.com

I leave you now with my prayer that you are able to find the music inside of you and that you choose to play it with a finely-tuned Hormone Symphony.

In peace and good health and in the love of a merciful, loving, powerful, and brilliant God THE MASTER COMPOSER,

and please, whatever you do, don't die with the music still inside of you.

Sincerely,

Angeli Maun Akey, MD

Ad majorem Dei gloriam

Ageless Medical Solutions, LlC
6228 NW 43rd Street, Suite A
Gainesville, FL 32653
Phone: (352) 332-4640
Fax: (352) 332-6604
www.agelessmedicalsolutions.com

Glossary

Celiac Disease Antibody Titer
Antibodies are produced by the immune system in response to substances that the body perceives as threatening. The measurement of the amount of these antibodies is called a **titer**. The higher the antibody measurement or titer, the more the inflammation, which means higher disease activity. In celiac disease and in gluten sensitivity, the antibodies attack parts of the gluten protein; this "battle" causes a lot of inflammation (destruction). We look for evidence of this inflammation in these antibodies called anti-tissue transglutaminase (anti-TTG), anti-endomysial antibodies (anti-EMA), and anti-gliadin antibodies in the diagnosis. The higher the levels of the titers, the more it supports the diagnosis of celiac disease.

EMDR: Eye Movement Desensitization and Reprocessing
Patients who have suffered from trauma that produces effects like insomnia, nightmares, anxiety, or recurrent painful flashbacks can find relief in EMDR. It has been useful in recovery from traumatic incidents, sexual abuse, depression, panic attacks, eating disorders, poor self-image, stress, worry, performance anxiety, eating disorders and phobias. The American Psychiatric Association found EMDR to be effective in treatment of trauma and included it in their 2004 practice guideline. The Department of Veterans' Affairs and the Department of Defense included it in their clinical practice guideline in 2010 for the management of post-traumatic stress and "strongly recommended" EMDR.

Estradiol is the main female hormone providing feminizing effects such as breasts, vaginal lubrication, and abdominal fat. It is critical in bone health and maintains cardiovascular health in premenopausal women and has favorable effects on cholesterol, primarily raising the good cholesterol, HDL.

Functional foods are defined as being consumed as part of a usual diet but are demonstrated to have physiological benefits and/or reduce the risk of chronic disease beyond basic nutritional functions.

High Intensity Interval Training (HIIT) is a type of cardiopulmonary training that uses short spurts of maximal intensity exercise to burn abdominal fat at rest. For example if maximal heart intensity is 220 minus your age, then for short durations of 30 seconds to 2 minutes one is to exercise at this maximal intensity with rests of 2 minutes in between. Numerous studies have documented the efficiency of this type of exercise at burning fat at rest as it increases basal metabolic rate and makes the fat burning furnaces more efficient in the body (see Appendix A).

Insulin is the hormone that is important in managing blood sugar. High circulating insulin levels are associated with oxidative stress to tissues, however. Oxidative stress is corrosive to tissue like rust is to metal.

Low Glycemic Index Diet is a type of eating that encourages foods that do not spike the blood sugar so that the insulin is not high. I call this "taming the insulin –glucose curves". This is useful in shrinking abdominal fat.

Nutraceutical, a portmanteau of nutrition and pharmaceutical, refers to extracts of foods claimed to have a medicinal effect on human health. The nutraceutical is usually contained in a medicinal format such as a capsule, tablet or powder in a prescribed dose. More rigorously, nutraceutical implies that the extract or food is demonstrated to have a physiological benefit or provide protection against a chronic disease.

Progesterone is the second female hormone which tends to decrease proportionally in a woman's body after the age of 35. It is present on every cell in a woman's body including the brain, heart, and uterus. As it acts on the same receptors as such calming medications as Valium™ and alcoholic beverages, when its levels go down (usually after age 35 around the second half of menstrual cycles), a woman tends to be anxious and have insomnia. I find it useful to give topically in the second half of the menstrual cycle to treat PMS symptoms.

Testosterone (also known as androgen) is primarily a male hormone, but is also important to women. It provides the virilizing effects in men. It increases lean body mass and strengthens memory and mental tenacity and provides for libido in both men and women. It is also important on bone health. More and more research evidence is showing testosterone is important in the health of women too (Davis, 2008).

Appendix

Appendix A

HIGH INTENSITY INTERVAL TRAINING (HIIT)

Workout time: 4 cycles, up to 16 minutes
Exercise: walk/run/swim, treadmill, stationary bicycle, Stairmaster/elliptical

Beginner – Perform 3 days per week: walk, treadmill, or bike

#1 cycle = 4 min	#2 cycle = 4 min	#3 cycle = 4 min	#4 cycle = 16 min
2 min – 2 min (mild) – (mod)	2 min – 2 min (mild) – (mod)	2 min – 2 min (mild) – (mod)	2 min – 2 min (mild) – (mod)

- 2 minute *mild* pace = fast grocery shopping
- 2 minute *moderate* pace = break a sweat up to 2 minutes

Intermediate – Perform 4 days per week: walk/run, treadmill, bike, or swim – <u>Clear with Doctor</u>

#1 cycle = 4 min	#2 cycle = 4 min	#3 cycle = 4 min	#4 cycle = 16 min
2 min – 2 min (mild/mod) – (mod/int)	2 min – 2 min (mild/mod) – (mod/int)	2 min – 2 min (mild/mod) – (mod/int)	2 min – 2 min (mild/mod) – (mod/int)

- 2 minute *mild to moderate* pace = normal exercise
- 2 minute *moderate* pace = rapid heart rate (HR), breathless up to 2 minutes

Advanced – Perform 4 days per week: walk/run, treadmill, bike, and swim – <u>Clear with Doctor</u>

#1 cycle = 4 min	#2 cycle = 4 min	#3 cycle = 4 min	#4 cycle = 16 min
2 min – 2 min (mod) – (max)	2 min – 2 min (mod) – (max)	2 min – 2 min (mod) – (max)	2 min – 2 min (mod) – (max)

- 2 minute *moderate* pace = rapid HR, breathless
- 2 minute *max* pace = max HR, breathless

* Repeat your second set increasing your intensity as tolerated. If you want to ramp up the challenge, increase the *amount of time* you walk, etc. at the *faster speed*. If you don't feel like that increase is giving you a challenge, go up a notch until you've increased your speed by 20 to 25%, then hold that speed and maintain it for up to 2 minutes. If you can do it for up to 2 minutes, great; if not, don't worry! It is more important to simply *follow this pattern*. Ideally, while in your HIIT mode, you should feel winded and unable to hold a conversation.

* Add strength training *up to 3 times per week*, whether at the gym or home. Home exercise might include: free weights, bench press, push-ups, wall squats, and sit-ups. It ideally targets all large muscle groups (i.e. arms, legs, chest, back, buttocks, and abdomen). For further reference: http://www.alsearsmd.com/

Appendix B

Average Testosterone Levels by Age in Men

Measurements in Conventional Units **(ng/dl)**, SHBG in (nmol/L)

Age	Number of Subjects	Total Test	Stand. Dev.	Free Test	Stand. Dev.	SHBG	Stand. Dev.
25-34	45	617	170	12.3	2.8	35.5	8.8
35-44	22	668	212	10.3	1.2	40.1	7.9
45-54	23	606	213	9.1	2.2	44.6	8.2
55-64	43	562	195	8.3	2.1	45.5	8.8
65-74	47	524	197	6.9	2.3	48.7	14.2
75-84	48	471	169	6.0	2.3	51.0	22.7
85-100	21	376	134	5.4	2.3	65.9	22.8

Vermeulen, A. (1996). *Declining Androgens with Age: An Overview.*

Measurements in Conventional Units **(ng/dl)**

Age	Number of Subjects	Mean Total Test	Stand. Dev.	Median Total Test	5th %	10th %	95th %
<25	125	692	158	697	408	468	956
25-29	354	669	206	637	388	438	1005
30-34	330	621	194	597	348	388	975
35-39	212	597	189	567	329	388	945
40-44	148	597	198	597	319	378	936
45-49	154	546	163	527	329	358	846
50-54	164	544	187	518	289	348	936
55-59	155	552	174	547	319	338	866

Simon, D., Nahoul, K., & Charles M.A. (1996). *Sex Hormones, Aging, Ethnicity and Insulin Sensitivity in Men: An Overview of the TELECOM Study.*

Bibliography

23 and me. Retrieved October 16, 2011, from www.23andme.com.

Angell, Marcia. (2005). *The Truth About the Drug Companies: How They Deceive Us and What to Do About It.* Random House Trade Paperbacks.

Atwood, C. S. (2005). Dysregulation of the Hypothalamic-Pituitary-Gonadal Axis with Menopause and Andropause Promotes Neurodegenerative Senescence. *J. Neuropathol. Exp. Neurol., 64* (2), 93-103.

Bach, Richard. (1970). *Jonathan Livingston Seagull.*

Belmaker, R. (2008). Mechanisms of Disease: Major Depressive Disorder. *New England Journal of Medicine, 358,* 55-68.

Bi, Yufang. (2011). Relationship of Urinary Bisphenol A Concentration to Risk for Prevalent Type 2 Diabetes in Chinese Adults: A Cross-sectional Analysis, *155*:368-374.

Bloss, C., Schork, N., & Topol, E. (2011). Effect of Direct-to-Consumer Genomewide Profiling to Assess Disease Risk. *New England Journal of Medicine, 364,* 524-534.

Braverman, Eric. (2007). *Younger You.* McGraw-Hill Books, NY.

Brent, G. (2008). Mechanisms of Disease: Grave's Disease. *New England Journal of Medicine, 358,* 2594-2605.

Catassi, Carlo, F. A. (2010). Celiac Disease Diagnosis: Simple Rules are Better than Complicated Algorithms. *The American Journal of Medicine, 123*(8), 691-693.

Cherrier, M. (2005). Testosterone Improves Spacial Memory in Men with Alzheimer's Disease and Mild Cognitive Impairment. *Neurology,* 2063-2068.

Davis S.R., et. al. (2008). Testosterone for Low Libido in Postmenopausal Women Not Taking Estrogen. *New England Journal of Medicine 359,* 2005 – 2017.

Deutsch, R., and Rivera, R. (2002). *Your Hidden Food Allergies are Making You Fat.* Prima Publishing.

Diamanti-Kandarakis, E. et al. (2009). Endocrine-Disrupting Chemicals: An Endocrine Society Scientific Statement. *Endocrine Reviews 30*(4):293-342.

Green, Peter. (2007). Medical progress: Celiac Disease. *The New England Journal of Medicine, 357*:1731-1740.

Esselstyn, C. B. (2007). *Prevent and Reverse Heart Disease.* New York, NY: Penguin Group.

Files, Julia. (2011). Bioidentical Hormone Therapy. *Mayo Clinic Proceedings. 86*(7):673-680.

Holick, MF. (2007). Vitamin D Deficiency. *New England Journal of Medicine. 357*:266-281.

Lane, R. E. (2010). Diabetes-Associated SorCS1 Regulates Alzheimer's Amyloid-Beta Metabolism: Evidence for Involvement of SorL1 and the Retromer Complex. *The Journal of Neuroscience, 30* (39), 13110-13115.

Lee, J. (2006). *Dr. John Lee's Hormone Balance Made Simple.* New York, NY: Warner Books.

Moberg, K. U. (2003). *The Oxytocin Factor: Tapping the Hormone of Calm, Love, and Healing.* Cambridge, Mass: Da Capo Press.

Moffat, S. (2004). Free testosterone and risk for Alzheimer's disease in older men. *Neurology, 62*, 188-193.

Muller, M. (2005). Endogenous Sex Hormones and Metabolic Syndrome in Aging Men. *Journal of Clinical Endocrinology and Metabolism, 90*, 2618-2623.

Nejad M., et. al. (2011). Subclincial celiac disease and gluten sensitivity. *Gastroenterology and Hepatology from Bed to Bench, 4*(3), 102-108.

Nelson, L. M. (2009). Primary Ovarian Insufficiency. *New England Journal of Medicine, 360*, 606-614.

Ohara, T., et. al. (2011). Glucose tolerance status and risk of dementia in the community: The Hisayama Study. *Neurology, 77*, 1126-1134.

Peck, M. S. (1978). *The Road Less Traveled.* New York, NY, USA: Simon and Schuster.

Powell, J. (1974). *The Secret of Staying in Love.* Argus Communications books.

Powell, J. (1978). *Unconditional Love.* Argus Communications Books.

Powell, J. (1967). *Why Am I Afraid to Love?* Argus Communications Books.

Powell, J. (1969). *Why Am I Afraid to Tell You Who I Am.* Argus Communications Books.

Practice Committee of the American Society for Reproductive Medicine. (2004). Current evaluation of amenorrhea. *Fertil Steril, 82* (Supp 1), S33-S39.

Rahman, A. (2008). Mechanisms of Disease: Systemic Lupus Erythematosus. *New England Journal of Medicine, 358*, 929-939.

Rhoden, E. (2004). Risks of Testosterone-Replacement Therapy and Recommendations for Monitoring. *New England Journal of Medicine*, 482-491.

Sacks, Frank, et. al. (2009). Comparison of Weight-Loss Diets with Different Compositions of Fat, Protein, and Carbohydrates. *New England Journal of Medicine, 360*, 859-873.

Simon, D., Nahoul, K., & Charles M.A. (1996). Sex Hormones, Aging, Ethnicity and Insulin Sensitivity in Men: An Overview of the TELECOM Study. *Androgens and the Aging Male* (p. 85-102). New York: Parthenon Publishing.

Spiegel, K., et. al. (2004). Sleep Duration and Levels of Hormones That Influence Hunger. *Annals of Internal Medicine, 141*, 846-850.

Stazi AV, M. A. (2000). A risk factor for female fertility and pregnancy: celiac disease. *Gynecol Endocrinol, 14*, 454-463.

Tancredi, A. (2004). Interest of Androgen Deficiency in Aging Males (ADAM) questionnaire for the identification of hypogonadism in elderly community dwelling male volunteers. *European Journal of Endocrinology, 151*, 355-360.

Travison, T. G. (2006). The Relative Contributions of Aging, Health, and Lifestyle Factors to Serum Testosterone Decline in Men. *The Journal of Clinical Endocrinology and Metabolism, 92*, 549-555.

Tarakanov A.V., Grinberg I.Z., Milyutina N.P. (2003). Universal mechanisms of SCENAR-effect in oxidative stress. *Reflexotherapy*; 4 (7), 41-45.

Vermeulen, A. (1996). Declining Androgens with Age: An Overview. *Androgens and the Aging Male* (pp. 3-14). New York: Parthenon Publishing.

Wang, L., McLeod, H., & Weinshelbaum, R. (2011). Genomic Medicine: Genomics and Drug Response. *New England Journal of Medicine, 364*, 1144-50.

Wilder, Laura Ingalls. (1932). *Little House on the Prairie.*

Young, William Paul. (2008). *The Shack.* Windblown Media Publishing.

About the Author

Angeli Maun Akey MD, FACP, ABAARM is board certified in internal medicine and anti-aging and regenerative medicine and has been in clinical practice for over fifteen years. She comes from a family of physicians and was born in Elizabeth, New Jersey. She grew up in Gainesville, Florida, where her mother, a physician, took a position at the University of Florida's Student Health Care Center (where she still practices at age 72!).

At the age of 16, Dr. Akey entered the University of Florida (UF) with five academic and music scholarships. At age 18, she was one of seven selected to the accelerated Junior Honors Medical Program making her the youngest ever accepted into the UF College of Medicine.

That same year, she placed in the top ten in the Miss Teen of America scholarship pageant and was inaugurated into the UF Hall of Fame.

She graduated Phi Beta Kappa with a BA in music (vocal performance), and a BS in interdisciplinary basic biological and medical sciences.

Because of her interest in public health and health policy, Dr. Akey joined the U.S. Public Health Service in medical school and was commissioned an Ensign. This led her to a rotation with the U.S. Surgeon General, Dr. Antonia Novello, who encouraged her to go into primary care.

Shortly after her 23rd birthday, she graduated from UF medical school with Alpha Omega Alpha distinction. She then completed her internship and residency in internal medicine at Yale-New Haven Hospital in Connecticut.

In 1996, she joined the Yale School of Medicine clinical faculty as Chief Medical Resident at the Hospital of St. Raphael, an affiliated hospital.

In 1997, she was recruited to start Harvard's Massachusetts General Hospital – affiliated Palm Beach Institute of Preventive Medicine. At the request of her high-profile patients, it was at this time she studied and learned to prescribe bioidentical hormones. She practiced in Palm Beach, Florida until the birth of her first son after a complicated pregnancy in 1999. At that time, she and her husband, Tim, decided to move back home to Gainesville.

Dr. Akey was a hospitalist physician for five years while simultaneously growing her private outpatient practice, North Florida Internal Medicine, which opened in 2000. In addition, her interest in other healing traditions led her to teach at the Florida School of Acupuncture and Oriental Medicine and the Dragon Rises School of Acupuncture and Oriental Medicine. In 2002, seeing where the future of medicine was headed, she opened Ageless Medical Solutions, a wellness and preventive practice that incorporates extensive complementary and alternative medicine (CAM).

She now specializes in detection of chronic diseases at their earliest stages and slowing down or reversing the process. As a courtesy Clinical Assistant Professor of Medicine at the UF College of Medicine, she enjoys teaching her holistic approach to pharmacy students, medical students, medical residents and other doctors in her office.

She is an avid reader in her search for Truth, and her other hobbies include singing and playing the piano; training in Krav Maga (Israeli-style martial arts) with her boys, Timothy Jr. and Derek, and her husband, Tim; traveling to Rome and learning Italian; and running with her Golden Retriever, Trooper.

She finds no compatibility issues between faith and science and looks to Blessed Pope John Paul II's writings on faith and reason for guidance, and especially likes what another of her intellectual mentors has said:

"My religion consists of a humble admiration of the illimitable superior spirit who reveals himself in the slight details we are able to perceive with our frail and feeble minds. That deeply emotional conviction of the presence of a superior reasoning power, which is revealed in the incomprehensible universe, forms my idea of God."
 --Albert Einstein